FIRST AID FOR THE®

OBSTETRICS & GYNECOLOGY BOARDS

JEANNINE RAHIMIAN, MD, MBA

Chief, Generalist Division
Department of Obstetrics and Gynecology
David Geffen School of Medicine at University of California, Los Angeles
Los Angeles, California

Series Editor

TAO T. LE, MD, MHS

Chief, Section of Allergy and Immunology
Department of Medicine
University of Louisville School of Medicine
Louisville, Kentucky

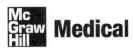 **Medical**

New York / Chicago / San Francisco / Lisbon / London / Madrid / Mexico City
Milan / New Delhi / San Juan / Seoul / Singapore / Sydney / Toronto

The McGraw·Hill Companies

First Aid for the® Obstetrics & Gynecology Boards

1 2 3 4 5 6 7 8 9 0   QPD/QPD   0 9 8 7 6

ISBN-13: 978-0-07-145531-2
ISBN-10: 0-07-145531-0

This book is printed on acid-free paper.

This book was set in Palatino by International Typesetting and Composition.
The editors were Catherine Johnson and Christie Naglieri.
The production supervisor was Phil Galea.
Project management was provided by International Typesetting and Composition.
Quebecor World Dubuque was printer and binder.

NOTICE

Library of Congress Cataloging-in-Publication Data

Rahimian, Jeannine.
    First aid for the obstetrics and gynecology boards / Jeannine Rahimian.—1st ed.
        p. ; cm.
    Includes index.
    ISBN 0-07-145531-0 (softcover)
    1. Obstetrics—Examinations, questions, etc.   2. Gynecology—Examinations, questions, etc.   I. Title.
    [DNLM: 1. Obstetrics—Examination Questions.   2. Gynecology—Examination Questions. WQ 18.2 R147   2006]
    RG111.R34   2006
    618.0076—dc22   2006048216

INTERNATIONAL EDITION ISBN-13: 978-0-07-110086-1; ISBN-10: 0-07-110086-5
Copyright © 2007. Exclusive rights by The McGraw-Hill Companies, Inc., for manufacture and export. This book cannot be re-exported from the country to which it is consigned by McGraw-Hill. The International Edition is not available in North America.

DEDICATION

To our families, friends, and loved ones, who supported us in the task of assembling this guide.

and

To the contributors to this and future editions, who took time to share their knowledge, insight, and humor for the benefit of residents and clinicians.

CONTENTS

CONTRIBUTORS

Gayane Ambartsymyan, MD

Assistant Clinical Professor
David Geffen School of Medicine
University of California, Los Angeles
Los Angeles, California

Malika Amneus, MD

Department of Obstetrics and Gynecology
David Geffen School of Medicine
University of California, Los Angeles
Los Angeles, California

Malini Anand, MD

Department of Obstetrics and Gynecology
David Geffen School of Medicine
University of California, Los Angeles
Los Angeles, California

Caroline M. Colin, MD, MS

Department of Obstetrics and Gynecology
David Geffen School of Medicine
University of California, Los Angeles
Los Angeles, California

Julie Henriksen, MD, FACOG

Assistant Professor
Department of Obstetrics and Gynecology
David Geffen School of Medicine
University of California, Los Angeles
Los Angeles, California

Chai Lin Hsu, MD

The Doctor's Office for Women
Newport Beach, California

Susan Huser, CNM, MS, FACNM

Nurse-Midwife
Department of Obstetrics and Gynecology
University of California, Los Angeles
Los Angeles, California

Daniel A. Kahn, MD, PhD

Chief Resident
Department of Obstetrics and Gynecology
David Geffen School of Medicine
University of California, Los Angeles
Los Angeles, California

Linda A. Lewis, MD

Department of Obstetrics and Gynecology
David Geffen School of Medicine
University of California, Los Angeles
Los Angeles, California

Judith A. Mikacich, MD

Assistant Professor
Department of Obstetrics and Gynecology
David Geffen School of Medicine
University of California, Los Angeles
Los Angeles, California

Susan Sarajari, MD, PhD

Fellow, Division of Reproductive Endocrinology and Infertility
Department of Obstetrics and Gynecology
David Geffen School of Medicine
University of California, Los Angeles
Los Angeles, California

Jill Satorie, MD

Assistant Clinical Professor
Department of Obstetrics and Gynecology
David Geffen School of Medicine
University of California, Los Angeles
Los Angeles, California

Jessica Spencer, MD

Fellow, Division of Reproductive Endocrinology and Infertility
Department of Gynecology and Obstetrics
Emory University
Atlanta, Georgia

Anita Trudell, CNM, MSN

Department of Obstetrics and Gynecology
David Geffen School of Medicine
University of California, Los Angeles
Los Angeles, California

Mor Tzadik, MD, MS

Department of Obstetrics and Gynecology
David Geffen School of Medicine
University of California, Los Angeles
Los Angeles, California

Milena M. Weinstein, MD

Fellow, Division of Urogynecology and Pelvic Reconstructive Medicine
Department of Reproductive Medicine
University of California, San Diego
San Diego, California

FACULTY REVIEWERS

Jonathan S. Berek, MS, MMS
Professor and Chair
Department of Obstetrics and Gynecology
Stanford University School of Medicine
Stanford, California

Brian J. Koos, MD, DPhil
Professor and Vice Chair, Academic Affairs
Department of Obstetrics and Gynecology
David Geffen School of Medicine
University of California, Los Angeles
Los Angeles, California

Alan H. DeCherney, MD
Branch Chief
Reproductive Biology and Medicine Branch
National Institute of Child Health and Development
Bethesda, Maryland

Linda W. Shiue, MD
Assistant Clinical Professor
Department of Medicine
University of California, San Francisco
San Francisco, California

PREFACE

With *First Aid for the Obstetrics & Gynecology Boards*, we hope to provide residents and clinicians with the most useful and up-to-date preparation guide for the American Board of Obstetrics and Gynecology (ABOG) certification and recertification exams. This new addition to the *First Aid* series represents an outstanding effort by a talented group of authors and includes the following:

- A practical exam preparation guide with resident-tested and study strategies
- Concise summaries of thousands of board-tested topics
- High-yield tables, diagrams, and illustrations
- Key facts in the margins highlighting *must know* information for the boards
- Mnemonics throughout, making learning memorable and fun

We invite you to share your thoughts and ideas to help us improve *First Aid for the Obstetrics & Gynecology Boards*. See How to Contribute, p. xv.

Los Angeles	Jeannine Rahimian
Louisville	Tao T. Le

ACKNOWLEDGMENTS

This has been a collaborative project from the start. We gratefully acknowledge the thoughtful comments, corrections, and advice of the residents and faculty who have supported the authors in the development of *First Aid for the Obstetrics & Gynecology Boards*.

For support and encouragement throughout the process, we are grateful to Nouzhan Sehati and Thao Pham.

Thanks to our publisher, McGraw-Hill, for the valuable assistance of their staff. For enthusiasm, support, and commitment to this challenging project, thanks to our editor, Catherine Johnson. A special thanks to International Typesetting and Composition for remarkable production work.

Our apologies if we accidentally omitted or misspelled your name.

Los Angeles   Jeannine Rahimian
Louisville   Tao T. Le

HOW TO CONTRIBUTE

To continue to produce a high-yield review source for the ABOG exam, you are invited to submit any suggestions or corrections. We also offer *paid internships* in medical education and publishing ranging from 3 months to 1 year (see next page for details). Please send us your suggestions for:

- Study and test-taking strategies for the ABOG
- New facts, mnemonics, diagrams, and illustrations
- Low-yield topics to remove

For each entry incorporated into the next edition, you will receive a $10 gift certificate, as well as personal acknowledgment in the next edition. Diagrams, tables, partial entries, updates, corrections, and study hints are also appreciated, and significant contributions will be compensated at the discretion of the authors. Also let us know about material in this edition that you feel is low yield and should be deleted.

The preferred way to submit entries, suggestions, or corrections is via electronic mail. Please include name, address, institutional affiliation, phone number, and e-mail address (if different from the address of origin). If there are multiple entries, please consolidate into a single e-mail or file attachment. Please send submissions to:

firstaidteam@yahoo.com

Otherwise, please send entries, neatly written or typed on a disk (Microsoft Word), to:

First Aid Team
914 N. Dixie Avenue, Suite 100
Elizabethtown, KY 42701

NOTE TO CONTRIBUTORS

All entries become property of the authors and are subject to editing and reviewing. Please verify all data and spellings carefully. In the event that similar or duplicate entries are received, only the first entry received will be used. Include a reference to a standard textbook to facilitate verification of the fact. Please follow the style, punctuation, and format of this edition if possible.

INTERNSHIP OPPORTUNITIES

The author team is pleased to offer part-time and full-time paid internships in medical education and publishing to motivated medical students and physicians. Internships may range from 3 months (e.g., a summer) up to a full year. Participants will have the opportunity to author, edit, and earn academic credit on a wide variety of projects, including the popular *First Aid* series. Writing and editing experience, familiarity with Microsoft Word, and Internet access are desired. For more information, e-mail a resume or a short description of your experience along with a cover letter to

firstaidteam@yahoo.com

CHAPTER 1

Introduction: Guide to the ABOG Exam

Jeannine Rahimian, MD, MBA

How Do I Register to Take the Exam?

You can register for the exam by going to the "Certification" section at www.abog.org. A written request for an application must be made to ABOG. The Board can be contacted via one of the following methods:

The American Board of Obstetrics and Gynecology
2915 Vine Street
Dallas, TX 75204
Phone: (214) 871-1619
Fax: (214) 871-1943
Email: info@abog.org

Registration Fees and Deadlines

The deadline for request of an application is usually November of the year just prior to taking the June examination (always the last Monday in June). The application fee is around $700 and there is an additional late fee of $315 for late applications. Check the ABOG website for the latest registration deadlines, fees, and policies.

How is the ABOG Examination Structured?

The ABOG written examination is a one half day paper based test administered at test centers across the country. The examination consists of objective, single best answer, multiple choice questions. According to the Board, the questions contain a continuum of answers, such that all possible answers may be correct, but only one answer is the **most** correct.

What Topics are Covered in the Examination?

Question content is based on a "blueprint" developed by the ABOG, which can be reviewed in the General Bulletin found in the downloads section of the website at www.abog.org. Approximately 30% of the questions are topics listed under gynecology, 30% are from the topics listed under obstetrics and 30% are from the topics listed under office practice. The remaining 10% of questions are based on cross-content topics, such as genetics, immunology and pharmacology. The website includes a list of major areas of emphasis.

The good news about the ABOG written examination is that it tends to focus on the diagnosis and management of diseases and conditions that you have likely seen as a resident and that you should expect to see as an obstetrician gynecologist specialist. *First Aid* and a good source of practice questions may be all you need to study for the exam. However, you should consider using standard textbooks to refer to topics for which you may need a more in depth review.

Ideally, you should start your preparation in the second half of your last year of residency. As you study, concentrate on the common diseases, learning both common and uncommon presentations. For uncommon diseases, focus on the classic presentations and manifestations. Draw on your experiences of residency training to anchor some of your learning. When you take the exam, you will realize that you've seen most of the clinical scenarios in your four years of rotations, clinics, case conferences, or grand rounds.

▶ TEST TAKING ADVICE

By this point in your life, you've probably gained much in the way of test-taking experience. Here are a few tips to keep in mind:

- For the long vignette questions, read the question stem and scan the options, then go back and read the case. You may get your answer without having to read through the whole case.
- There is no penalty for guessing, so you should **never** leave a question blank.
- Good **pacing** is very important. Make sure to leave adequate time to get to all the questions. On average, you have approximately one minute per question, so if you don't know the answer within a short period, make an educated guess and move on.
- It's fine to **second guess** yourself. Research shows that our second hunches tend to be better than our first guesses.
- Don't panic with "impossible" questions. They may be **experimental** questions that won't count.
- Note the age and race of the patient. When ethnicity is given, it may be relevant.

CHAPTER 2

Obstetrics

Jeannine Rahimian, MD, MBA
Julie Henriksen, MD, FACOG
Jill Satorie, MD
Mor Tzadik, MD, MS
Judith A. Mikacich, MD
Jessica Spencer, MD
Chai Lin Hsu, MD
Susan Huser, CNM, MS, FACNM
Anita Trudell, CNM, MSN

Gametogenesis

- Formation of haploid gametes (sperm and oocytes) is via meiosis.
- Female germ cells (oogonia):
  - Migrate to genital ridge at 7 weeks gestation.
  - Reach maximum of 6 million at 20 weeks gestation.
  - Enter and stay in meiosis prophase I and are then called **oocytes.**
- By the time of birth, there are 1–2 million oocytes.
- During ovulation, oocytes progress from meiosis I to meiosis II.
- Completion of meiosis II requires fertilization.

The number of oocytes in the female gonad peaks at 20 weeks of gestation.

Fertilization

- Egg and sperm usually meet in ampulla of fallopian tube (Figure 2-1).
- The sperm penetrates the zona pellucida and is engulfed by vitelline membrane.
- When sperm chromatin enters egg cytoplasm:
  - Male pronucleus is formed.
  - Oocyte completes meiosis II, resulting in female pronucleus.
- A **zygote** is the cell resulting from fertilization of female and male pronuclei.

Embryonic Development

SINGLETON

- Zygote undergoes **cleavage** (repetitive mitosis) into cells called **blastomeres** as it travels along the fallopian tube (Figure 2-1).

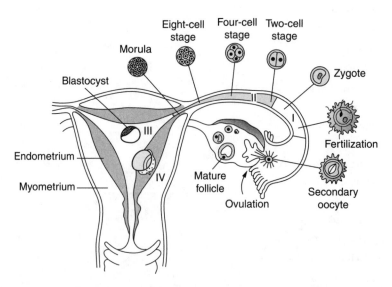

FIGURE 2–1. Diagrammatic summary of the ovarian cycle, fertilization, and human blastocyst development during the first week.

(Adapted with permission from Moore KL. *The Developing Human: Clinically Oriented Embryology*, 4th ed. Philadelphia, Saunders, 1988; Cunningham, et al. *Williams Obstetrics*, 21st ed. New York, NY: McGraw-Hill, 2001: 131, Fig. 7-1.)

- See Figure 2-2 for diagrams of various stages of cleavage.
- The **morula** (solid ball of 12–16 blastomeres) is formed day 3 after fertilization.
- Blastomeres separate into outer and inner cell mass, or **blastocyst**, at day 5.
- Outer cell mass:
  - Differentiates into cytotrophoblast and syncytiotrophoblast.
  - Eventually gives rise to the placenta.

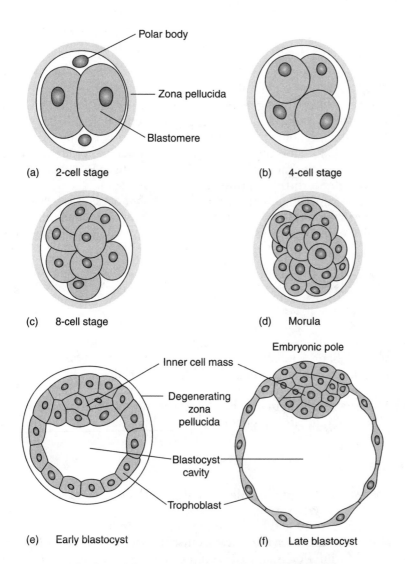

FIGURE 2–2. **Cleavage of the zygote and formation of the blastocyst.**

A to D show various stages of cleavage. The period of the morula begins at the 12- to 16-cell stage and ends when the blastocyst forms, which occurs when there are 50 to 60 blastomeres present. E and F are sections of blastocysts. The zona pellucida has disappeared by the late blastocyst stage (5 days). The polar bodies shown in A are small, nonfunctional cells that soon degenerate. (With permission from Moore KL. *The Developing Human: Clinically Oriented Embryology*, 4th ed. Philadelphia, Saunders, 1988; Cunningham, et al. *Williams Obstetrics*, 21st ed. New York, NY: McGraw-Hill, 2001:88, Fig. 5-2.)

- Inner cell mass develops into embryonic disc, then forming the primitive streak, notochord, and three germ layers, which are:
  - **Ectoderm** develops into epidermis, nervous system, pituitary gland.
  - **Mesoderm** develops into dermis, muscle, skeleton, urogenital system, gonads.
  - **Endoderm** develops into epithelium and glandular cells of respiratory and gastrointestinal tracts.
- **Embryonic period** (weeks 3–8 after fertilization): Major body structures develop.
- **Fetal period** (9 weeks after fertilization): Tissues and organs undergo differentiation and rapid fetal growth.

TWIN GESTATION

Diamniotic, dichorionic pregnancies can be either dizygotic or monozygotic.

- 2/3 of twin pregnancies are dizygotic.
- All dizygotic twins are diamniotic, dichorionic.
- Rate of dizygotic twinning increases with maternal age and is hereditary.
- Monozygotic twins have the following characteristics:
  - 1/3 diamniotic, dichorionic. Occurs if division is ≤72 hours after fertilization. (before morula differentiates into inner and outer cell mass).
  - 2/3 diamniotic, monochorionic. Occurs if division is between 4 and 8 days after fertilization (during blastocyst stage).
  - 1% monoamniotic, monochorionic. Occurs if division is between 8 and 13 days after fertilization (after chorion and amnion differentiate).
  - 1/1000 conjoined twins. Occurs if division is >13 days after fertilization.

▶ PHYSIOLOGY OF PREGNANCY

Genital Tract

- See Table 2-1 for genital tract changes during pregnancy.
- Abnormal changes include:
  - **Pregnancy luteoma**, benign solid tumor of ovary rarely associated with maternal and fetal virilization. Usually regress after delivery.
  - **Hyperreactio luteinalis**, benign cystic tumor, commonly associated with maternal virilization and very high hCG levels.

Cardiovascular

- List of changes to cardiovascular system is found in Table 2-2.
- 90% will have systolic murmurs.
- S1 split often heard and heart is often displaced to left.
- **Supine hypotensive syndrome,** occurs in 10%, is symptomatic hypotension due to inferior vena cava compression resulting in reduced cardiac preload.
- Total number of red blood cells increase, but concentration decreases due to greater increase in plasma volume, resulting in a **physiological anemia**.
- Hemoglobin of 12.5 is average at term, <11 considered abnormal.

Respiratory

- List of physiological respiratory changes is found in Table 2-3.
- Maternal oxygen consumption is increased.

TABLE 2-1. Genital Tract Changes During Pregnancy

Ovary	Corpus luteum secretes progesterone
Uterus	■ Increased size (from 70 to 1100 g) ■ Increased volume (from 10 mL to 5 L) ■ Leaves pelvis at 12 weeks, usually undergoes dextrorotation ■ Increase in nerves, blood flow, lymph ■ Hypertrophy of the fundus
Decidua (endometrium)	■ Thickens to 5–10 mm, mostly hypertrophy not hyperplasia ■ Decidua basalis: site of blastocyst implantation. Basal plate of placenta ■ Decidua capsularis: overlies the blastocyst ■ Decidua parietalis: lines the rest of the uterus
Cervix	■ Predominantly collagen, approximately 10% muscle fibers ■ Forms antimicrobial mucous plug during pregnancy ■ Blue appearance early, more red later with columnar epithelium eversion
Vagina	■ Copious acidic secretion is common ■ Lactobacillus concentrations higher ■ Chadwick sign: Violet color of vagina from hyperemia
Bony pelvis	■ Increased mobility of sacroiliac, sacrococcygeal, and pubic joints ■ Marked lordosis common

- Elevation of diaphragm displaces heart to the left, decreases functional residual capacity and residual volume.
- Hyperventilation results in physiological **respiratory alkalosis,** with decreased HCO_3^- (from 26 to 22 mmol/L) and mildly elevated pH.

Gastrointestinal

- Reflux is common due to delayed gastric emptying and decreased esophageal tone probably mediated by high progesterone and low motilin levels.
- Decrease in smooth muscle tone increases risk of aspiration and incidence of cholelithiasis.

TABLE 2-2. Cardiovascular Changes in Pregnancy

Heart rate	↑	Average increase of 10–15 beats per minute
Cardiac output	↑	Increases 30–50%
Blood volume	↑	Average of 40% (mostly between 10 and 20 weeks)
Vascular resistance	↓	Both pulmonic and systemic vascular resistance decrease
Colloid pressure	↓	Total albumin increased but *concentration* decreased

11

TABLE 2-3. **Respiratory Changes in Pregnancy**

Tidal volume and minute ventilation	↑↑
Minute O_2 uptake	↑
Respiratory rate	No change
Vital capacity	No change
Functional residual capacity	↓
Residual volume	↓

- The appendix often displaced upward and lateral toward right flank can result in atypical presentation of appendicitis.
- Alkaline phosphatase often elevated.

A displaced appendix can result in atypical presentation of appendicitis.

Weight Gain

- Average weight gain is 10–15 kg.
- 40% of gain due to fetus (~3400 g), amniotic fluid (~800 g), placenta (~650 g).
- 60% of gain distributed to maternal fat (~3,400 g), extravascular fluid (~1500 g), blood volume (~1500 g), uterine enlargement (~1000 g), breast enlargement (~400 g).

Urinary System

- See Table 2-4 for changes in the urinary system.
- Ureteral and renal dilation is common.
- Increased glomerular filtration rate can result in physiological glucosuria, decreased plasma levels of drugs excreted by kidney. Proteinuria is abnormal.

Thyroid

- List of thyroid hormone changes is found in Table 2-5.
- Elevated estrogen increases thyroxine binding globulin (TBG).

TABLE 2-4. **Changes to the Urinary System During Pregnancy**

Glomerular filtration rate (GFR)	↑ 50% Results in ↓ BUN and Cr
Bladder	Urinary tract infections and pyelonephritis more frequent
Renin-angiotensin-aldosterone axis	All ↑ in pregnancy Normal angiotensin II refractoriness not seen in preeclampsia

TABLE 2-5. Changes in Thyroid Hormones with Pregnancy

TBG	↑
Total T$_4$ and T$_3$	↑
Free T$_4$ and T$_3$	No change
TSH	↓ in first trimester

- Thyroid gland enlarges slightly, but rarely indicates abnormal thyroid function.

Skin and Hair

- Common skin changes are abdominal striae, chloasma (facial patches), melasma (mask of pregnancy).
- Linea nigra, areolae, and genital skin pigmentation mediated by melanocyte stimulating hormone. Usually regress after pregnancy.
- Pregnancy favors anagen (growth) phase of hair. Telogen (shedding) phase common during first 4 months postpartum.

Other Changes

- Increased intraocular pressure and corneal edema.
- Gums undergo vascular swelling known as **epulis of pregnancy**.
- Increased white blood cell count, but immunity is depressed.

▶ FETAL CIRCULATION

- Fetal component (chorionic villi) and maternal component (decidua basalis) of placenta are enclosed by cytotrophoblasts.
- Space between chorionic villi (intervillous space) is filled with blood from spiral arteries and is drained by endometrial veins.
- Villi contain blood vessels in a complex arteriocapillary-venous system providing a large exchange area for oxygen, carbon dioxide, nutrients, and waste products.
- Though small amounts of fetal blood can enter maternal circulation through defects, the placental villi (synciotrophoblast, cytotrophoblast, capillary wall) usually prevent mixing of fetal and maternal blood.
- Figure 2-3 is a schematic diagram of fetal circulation.
- Well-oxygenated blood goes into umbilical vein, which gives rise to ductus venosus.
- Oxygenated blood from ductus venosus flows preferentially through foramen ovale to left atrium and ventricle. Only a small amount of less oxygenated blood crosses the foramen ovale.
- Well-oxygenated blood in left ventricle is primarily distributed to the brain, myocardium, and upper body.
- Majority of less oxygenated blood in right ventricle passes through pulmonary artery to descending aorta via ductus arteriosus.

The placental villi separate maternal and fetal circulation, so there is no mixing of blood.

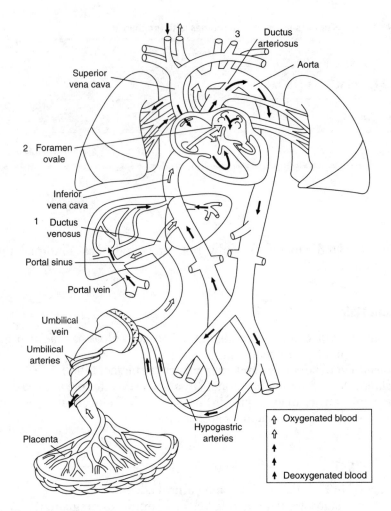

FIGURE 2–3. **Fetal circulation.**

(Reproduced, with permission, from Cunningham, et al. *Williams Obstetrics*, 21st ed. New York, NY: McGraw-Hill, 2001:144, Fig. 7-9)

> *Maternal alcohol use is the most preventable cause of birth defects in developed countries and is the most common cause of mental retardation.*

► **PRECONCEPTIONAL COUNSELING**

The goals of preconceptional counseling are to identify risk factors, improve pregnancy outcome, reduce obstetrical complications, and educate patients.

Current Health Status

OBESITY

- Overweight patients should be counseled on increased risks of gestational diabetes, preeclampsia, infertility.
- Weight reduction should be recommended.

SUBSTANCE ABUSE

- Maternal alcohol use is the most preventable cause of birth defects in developed countries and most common cause of mental retardation.
- Smoking is associated with low birth weight and other morbidities (see Prenatal Care section).

DIETARY CHANGES

- Limit caffeine intake <250 mg (4–5 cups of coffee) per day to optimize fertility and decrease risk of spontaneous abortion.
- High mercury-containing fish should be avoided (e.g., shark, swordfish, tilefish). Moderate mercury-containing fish (tuna) should be limited to 6 oz/week.
- Raw and undercooked meat should be avoided (toxoplasmosis risk).

IMMUNIZATIONS

- Rubella and varicella vaccination should be given if not immune.
- After immunization, should wait 1–3 months before attempting to conceive, although no teratogenic effects have been reported. Both are safe with breast-feeding.
- Nasal spray flu vaccine is live vaccine and should not be given during pregnancy.

PSYCHOSOCIAL STATUS

- Stress level, financial issues, domestic violence, social support, barriers to prenatal care, and work-related concerns should be assessed.

OTHER EXPOSURES

- Assess risk for occupational or household exposures.
- Avoidance of cat litter; gloves should be worn for gardening (toxoplasmosis risk).

Reproductive and Gynecological History

- Previous pregnancy outcomes and complications should be elicited.
- History of recurrent pregnancy loss, preeclampsia, intrauterine growth retardation, or fetal death should be reviewed, and appropriate treatment should be offered.
- Cervical cytology screening should be reviewed and treatment performed if needed.
- Sexually transmitted infections should be screened for and treated.

Medical History

CARDIAC DISEASE

- Maternal congenital heart disease:
  - Have increased risk of fetus with congenital heart disease (2–5% risk).
  - Should have cardiology and maternal fetal medicine evaluation before conception.
  - Hypertension should be well controlled and medications should be switched to those safe in pregnancy (e.g., methyldopa, labetalol).

ENDOCRINE DISORDERS

- Diabetes should be well controlled, switched to insulin if medication required, evaluated for nephropathy, and retinopathy before conception.
- Thyroid disorders should be well controlled before conception.

METABOLIC DISORDERS

- Women with phenylketonuria should adjust their diet to minimize phenylalanine level. High maternal levels (>20 mg/dL) can result in microcephaly, mental retardation, congenital heart disease, and intrauterine growth retardation.

EPILEPSY

- Epilepsy and antiseizure medications are associated with increased rate of malformations.
- Patients should be on lowest effective dose and least number of medications required.
- If seizures-free for ≥2 years, should discuss discontinuation of medication with neurologist.

THROMBOPHILIAS

- Consider aspirin and/or heparin therapy if indicated.

PSYCHIATRIC HISTORY

- Safer drug regimens, such as selective serotonin reuptake inhibitor or tricyclic antidepressants, should be initiated or substituted as needed.

Medications

- All women of childbearing age should take **folic acid** 0.4 mg/day to reduce risk of neural tube defects.
- Women with a previous child with a neural tube defect should take folic acid 4.0 mg/day for 3 months before attempting to conceive.
- Increased risk of neural tube defects also associated with:
    - Couples with sibling, niece, or nephew with a neural tube defect.
    - Women with Type 2 diabetes mellitus.
    - Women taking valproic acid or carbamazepine.
- Unnecessary medications, herbal supplements, and megavitamins should be discontinued or substituted to **prevent teratogenicity** (e.g., Coumadin, ACE inhibitors, Accutane).

Family History

Family history of these disorders warrants genetic counseling and/or testing:

- Multifactorial traits: Neural tube defect, congenital heart disease, cleft lip/palate.
- Inherited disorders: Muscular dystrophy, cystic fibrosis, Huntington chorea, hemophilia, kidney disease.
- Chromosomal abnormalities: Down syndrome, fragile X syndrome.
- Metabolic disorders: Diabetes mellitus, phenylketonuria.

Ethnicity

- Screening should be offered to those at risk (see Genetic Counseling section).

Laboratory Assessment

- All patients should have CBC with red cell indices, rubella titer, hepatitis B surface antigen, HIV, RPR, genital gonorrhea, and *chlamydia*.
- The following tests should be considered:
  - Varicella titer (if patient denies having had disease)
  - Hepatitis C antibody (high-risk populations)
  - TSH (if symptomatic or at risk)
  - Fasting blood sugar (family history of diabetes)
  - PPD (high-risk population)
  - Toxoplasmosis titer (if known exposure)
  - CMV titer (works in day care or dialysis units)
  - Genetic carrier screening (at risk secondary to family history or ethnicity)

▶ PRENATAL CARE

History

- Identify risk factors and determine appropriate intervention if needed (see Preconceptional Care section for standard history).

Physical Examination

- A thorough examination, including thyroid, heart, lung, and breast, to identify factors that could affect maternal or fetal outcome.
- Pelvic examination should include assessment of uterine size, cervical length, and dilation, and clinical pelvimetry.
- Uterine size discrepancy evaluated with pelvic ultrasound. Crown rump length measurement at 7–14 weeks is 95% accurate to within 3–5 days.
- Fetal heart tones heard with Doppler at 9–12 weeks.

Laboratory Tests

- Tests do not need repeating if normal values obtained at recent preconception visit.
- Routine prenatal labs may include:
  - Blood type, Rh type, antibody screen*
  - Hemoglobin and/or hematocrit*
  - Rubella antibody titer*
  - VDRL test*
  - Hepatitis B* surface antigen
  - Pap smear*
  - HIV*
  - Urine culture or urinalysis*
  - *Chlamydia* culture*
  - Gonorrhea culture
  - PPD (high-risk population)
  - Thyroid function (if symptomatic)

*Recommended by ACOG

- Additional tests at follow-up visits are: first trimester genetic screening at 11–13 weeks, second trimester screening (expanded maternal serum alpha fetoprotein [ms-AFP]) at 15–20 weeks, 1-hour glucose tolerance test at 24–28 weeks, hemoglobin and/or hematocrit at 28 weeks, and repeat third trimester sexually transmitted disease (STD) screening (if at risk).
- Risk factors for gestational diabetes are:
  - Advanced maternal age
  - High body mass index (BMI)
  - Family history
  - Prior macrosomic infant or gestational diabetes
  - Unexplained prior stillbirth
  - Non-Caucasian race

Follow-up Visits

- Rh negative patients should receive RhoGAM at 28 weeks, if father of baby is Rh positive.
- Fetal movement counting or "kick counts" should be started around 28 weeks.

Patient Education

NUTRITION

- Prenatal vitamins usually meet requirements for vitamins and minerals.
- Folic acid supplementation preconception and in early prenatal period shown to decrease the incidence of neural tube defects.
- Fish consumption and mercury content discussed (see Preconceptional Counseling section).
- Daily caffeine intake >500 mg increases risk of spontaneous abortion. May increase risk of stillbirth or decreased birth weight.

Recommended weight gain in pregnancy is based on prepregnancy Body Mass Index.

WEIGHT GAIN

- Recommended weight gain based on pre-pregnancy BMI (see Table 2-6).
- BMI is weight in kg divided by height in meters squared.

WORK

- A healthy woman with an uncomplicated pregnancy may work until onset of labor unless workplace results in potential hazard or risk of injury.

TABLE 2-6. **Recommended Weight Gain in Pregnancy**

BODY MASS INDEX	AVERAGE WEIGHT GAIN (LB)	AVERAGE WEIGHT GAIN (KG)
<19.8 (underweight)	28–40	12.5–18
19.8–26 (average weight)	25–35	11.5–16
>26 (overweight)	15–25	7–11.5

- Physically demanding work, prolonged standing, night work shown to be risk factors for preterm birth.
- Work should be limited or stopped in women with vaginal bleeding, pregnancy-induced hypertension, shortened cervix, fetal growth restriction, multiple gestation, polyhydramnios, or prior history of preterm birth.

EXERCISE

- Moderate exercise helps maintain cardiorespiratory and muscular fitness.
- Exercise of 20–30 minutes three times per week does not affect length of gestation or birth weight. Temporary increase in fetal heart rate baseline (5–15 bpm) during and shortly after exercise is common.
- Pregnant women should be cautioned regarding activities that increase risk of falls or excessive joint stress, such as skiing or jogging.
- Scuba diving and exertion in supine position should be advised against.
- Lifting weights is safe.
- Contraindications to aerobic exercise include:
  - Significant heart disease
  - Restrictive lung diseases
  - Multiple gestation at risk for premature labor
  - Persistent second/third trimester bleeding
  - Incompetent cervix/cerclage
  - Placenta previa (after 26 weeks)
  - Ruptured membranes
  - Preeclampsia or pregnancy induced hypertension

TRAVEL

- Airplane travel is safe in uncomplicated pregnancy. No increased risk of spontaneous abortions in air travelers.
- Women at risk for complications, such as preterm labor, pregnancy induced hypertension, and sickle cell disease, should not travel during pregnancy.

IMMUNIZATIONS

- Influenza vaccine should be given to all women pregnant during the flu season. The killed virus vaccine can be given in any trimester. The live vaccine (via nasal spray) should not be given to pregnant women.
- Hepatitis B series should be continued if started prior to conception and started for women at high risk for acquiring the infection.

SMOKING

- Smoking cessation conseling is important because smoking is associated with low birth weight, growth restriction, preterm delivery, preterm premature rupture of membranes, placental abruption, placenta previa, and sudden infant death syndrome.
- Secondhand smoke increases asthma, otitis media, and respiratory infections in children.
- Intensive counseling with pregnancy specific material, bupropion, and nicotine gum or patch are all accepted modalities in assisting with cessation.

Mendelian Disorders

- Single gene disorders are classified as autosomal or X linked, dominant or recessive. Disorders that can be diagnosed prenatally are included in parentheses.
- Ethnic groups at risk for heritable diseases are listed in Table 2-7.

AUTOSOMAL DOMINANT

- Typically have vertical transmission from one generation to next with males and females affected (e.g., neurofibromatosis, myotonic dystrophy, congenital adrenal hyperplasia, polycystic kidney disease, Huntington disease, osteogenesis imperfecta).
- **Penetrance** is the frequency a genotype results in a particular phenotype. Because of **variable penetrance**, not all individuals with an autosomal dominant mutation have affected parents.
- **Variable expression** is the range of phenotypic changes that can be exhibited with a particular genotype (differences in age of onset, severity of disease, and so forth).

TABLE 2-7. Ethnic Groups at Increased Risk for Heritable Diseases

ETHNIC GROUP	DISEASE	CARRIER RATE	RECOMMENDED SCREENING TEST
African American	Sickle cell (Hb SS)	1/12	Hb electrophoresis
	Sickle cell (Hb SC)	1/40	Hb electrophoresis
Asian	α thalassemia	1/5	MCV*
	β thalassemia	1/15	MCV*
Ashkenazi Jewish†	Tay-Sachs	1/30	Mutation analysis
	Cystic fibrosis	1/25	Mutation analysis
	Gaucher disease	1/15	Mutation analysis
	Familial dysautonomia	1/30	Mutation analysis
Mediterranean	α thalassemia	1/20	MCV*
	β thalassemia	1/10	MCV*
North European Caucasian	Cystic fibrosis	1/25	Mutation analysis
Native American	Cystic fibrosis	1/20	Mutation analysis

* Thalassemia should be screened with mean corpuscular volume (MCV). If MCV abnormal with normal iron studies, then check hemoglobin electrophoresis.

† Ashkenazi Jews also at risk for Bloom disease, Niemann-Pick, Fanconi anemia, Canavan disease.

AUTOSOMAL RECESSIVE

- Typically have two or more affected siblings (male and female) but no disease in parents or preceding generations (e.g., cystic fibrosis, phenylketonuria, Tay-Sachs).

X-LINKED DISEASES

- Only males are affected, females can be carriers. Typically see affected males in many generations (e.g., hemophilia A, Duchenne muscular dystrophy, fragile X).

Multifactorial Inheritance

- Do not follow mendelian inheritance pattern, but show evidence of genetic component.
- Due to combination of genetic and environmental factors. Common multifactorial traits include:
  - Cleft lip or palate
  - Congenital cardiac defects
  - Diaphragmatic hernia
  - Hydrocephalus
  - Mullerian fusion defects
  - Neural tube defects
  - Omphalocele
  - Posterior urethral valves
  - Pyloric stenosis
  - Renal agenesis
- If a single gene disorder, chromosome abnormality, or genetic syndrome ruled out, patients can be counseled regarding recurrence that:
  - Risk to siblings is higher than general population (1–5 %).
  - Risk is low for second degree relatives (<1%).
  - Risk is higher if >1 family member affected or if defect severe.

Aneuploidy

- Presence of incorrect number of chromosomes (e.g., 45 or 47). Trisomy 21, trisomy 13, trisomy 18, and monosomy X (Turner syndrome) are most common.
- Affects 3–4% of pregnancies and 1/160 live births.
- 50% of first trimester miscarriages due to aneuploidy as most are incompatible with life.
- Trisomy usually occurs due to error in maternal meiosis. Maternal age is most important risk factor.
- Most common **sex chromosome abnormalities** are 45X, 47XXY, 47XXX, 47XYY, and mosaicism, the presence of ≥2 cell populations with different karyotypes.
- Risk of second pregnancy with trisomy if one with trisomy 21, trisomy 18, trisomy 13, 47XXX, or 47XXY is 1% (or greater if >35 years old).

Structural Abnormalities

- Structural abnormalities include translocations, inversions, deletions, and duplications.

Approximately 50% of first trimester miscarriages are due to aneuploidy.

- Found on 1/2000 second trimester amniocenteses.
- **Translocation** is reciprocal exchange of genetic material between two nonhomologous chromosomes:
  - Balanced translocation, when no genetic material gained or lost, usually results in phenotypically normal individual. Found in 1/500 of phenotypically normal people.
  - If balanced translocation found on chorionic villus sampling or amniocentesis, parents should be tested. In 30%, one of parents carries translocation, which reassures that it is benign. *De novo* balanced translocation has 10–15% risk of fetal malformations.

Triploidy

- Triploidy, the presence of 69 chromosomes, occurs in 1–2% of recognized pregnancies and 15% of chromosomally abnormal aborted fetuses (see Gestational Trophoblastic Disease section).

Manifestations of Common Genetic Disorders

- Association between anomalies and aneuploidy risk is found in Table 2–8.
- Trisomy 21 (T21):
  - Variable degree of mental retardation.
  - Associated with characteristic facial features, duodenal atresia, tetralogy of Fallot.

TABLE 2–8. Major Anomalies and Associated Aneuploidy Risk

ANOMALY	RISK OF ANEUPLOIDY	MOST COMMON ANEUPLOIDY
Cystic hygroma	60–75%	45X, T21, T18, T13, XXY
Hydrops	30–80%	T13, T21, T18, 45X
Complete atrioventricular defect	40–70%	T21
Holoprosencephaly	40–60%	T13, T18
Omphalocele	30–40%	T13, T18
Duodenal atresia	20–30%	T21
Bladder outlet obstruction	20–25%	T13, T18
Diaphragmatic hernia	20–25%	T13, T18, T21, 45X
Cardiac defect	5–30%	T21, T18, T13, T22, T8, T9
Limb reduction	8%	T18
Club foot	6%	T18
Hydrocephalus	3–8%	T13, T18, triploidy

- Trisomy 13 (T13):
  - Little potential for extrauterine life.
  - Abnormalities usually detected with ultrasound (up to 95%).
  - Findings include **rocker bottom feet,** holoprosencephaly, midline facial defects, omphalocele, polydactyly, and club feet and hands.
- Trisomy 18 (T18):
  - Little potential for extrauterine life.
  - Abnormalities usually detected with ultrasound.
  - Findings include clenched hands, overlapping fourth digit, club foot, persistently extended legs, micrognathia, and congenital heart disease.
- Turner syndrome (monosomy X):
  - First trimester miscarriage occurs in 90% of affected pregnancies.
  - Usually have normal intelligence, ovarian failure, short stature, and a 20% incidence of heart malformations.

Genetic Counseling

Indications for genetic counseling include:
- Maternal age ≥35 before expected delivery
- Teratogen exposure during pregnancy
- Hereditary disease, birth defect, chromosomal abnormality or mental retardation in patient, previous child or family history
- Ethnic background with increased risk of heritable disease (see Table 2-7).
- ≥3 first trimester pregnancy loss
- Abnormal first or second trimester screening results
- ≥1 major anomaly detected on ultrasound

▶ OBSTETRIC SCREENING

Screening Tests

- All screening tests include ms-AFP. Values usually given as multiples of the median (MoM).
- Causes of abnormal ms-AFP levels listed in Table 2-9.
- Mean levels are higher in African Americans and lower in patients with insulin dependent diabetes mellitus.

FIRST TRIMESTER SCREENING

- At 11–13^6/$_7$ weeks.
- Screening for T21 and T18.
- **Method:** Measurement of serum free hCG and pregnancy-associated plasma protein-A (PAPP-A). Ultrasound measurement of nuchal translucency.
- **Results:** Free hCG ↑ in T21, ↓ in T18. PAPP-A ↓ in T21, ↓ in T18.
- **Accuracy:** Trisomy 21: 85% sensitive with 5% false positive rate, trisomy 18 : 91% sensitive with 2% false positive rate.
- **Management:** If abnormal, offer karyotype with chorionic villus sampling or amniocentesis. If negative, should still offer second trimester neural tube defect screening and anatomy survey.

EXPANDED MS-AFP (TRIPLE SCREEN)

- At 15–20 weeks.
- Screening for neural tube defects, T21 and T18.

TABLE 2-9. Causes of Abnormal Maternal Serum Alpha Fetoprotein

ELEVATED	DECREASED
Incorrect dates	Incorrect dates
Twins	Trisomy 21
Abruption	Obesity
Intrauterine death	
Neural tube defects	
Gastroschisis	
Chromosomal abnormalities	
Hydrops	

- **Method:** Immunoassay for ms-AFP, hCG, uE3 (unconjugated estriol).
- **Interpretation:** Higher false positive rate in women >35 years, but same sensitivity (see Table 2-10 for interpretation of triple screen results).
- **Quadruple screen** is expanded ms-AFP with addition of inhibin A.

Diagnostic Tests

CHORIONIC VILLUS SAMPLING

- At 11–14 weeks.
- Early chromosomal analysis.
- **Method:** Transcervical or transabdominal sampling of chorionic villi. RhoGAM given if patient Rh negative. Group B streptococcus, gonorrhea, and *Chlamydia* cultures should be done prior to procedure.
- **Accuracy:** 99% with 0.03% false positive rate.
- **Complications:** Fetal damage, fetal loss, mosaicism, bleeding, and infection. Early reports of limb reduction and cavernous hemangioma later showed no difference.

TABLE 2-10. Interpretation of Triple Screen Results

CONDITION	AFP	hCG	uE3
Down syndrome (69% detection rate)	↓	↑	↓
Trisomy 18 (60–75% detection rate)	↓	↓	↓
Open neural tube or abdominal wall defects (85% detection rate)	↑	n/a	n/a

AMNIOCENTESIS

- At 15–18 weeks.
- Chromosomal analysis, genetics studies, assessment of neural tube defects.
- Early amniocentesis <15 weeks has increased fetal loss and complications.
- **Method:** Amniotic fluid evaluated for AFP and chromosome analysis. RhoGAM given if patient Rh negative.
- **Accuracy:** >99%.
- **Complications:** Fetal injury, fetal death (most often in first 3 weeks), infection, bleeding, and rupture of membranes.

▶ ANTEPARTUM FETAL MONITORING

Non-Stress Test (NST)

- Measurement of amniotic fluid index (AFI) and fetal heart tracing for 20 minutes.
- Interpretation: Two accelerations of ≥15 bpm for ≥15 seconds. AFI with one pocket >2 cm or total of >6 cm over four quadrants.
- Indications: Decreased fetal movement ≥28 weeks, gestational diabetes, multiple gestation, preeclampsia, intrauterine growth restriction, fetal anomalies.
- Contraindications: None.

Contraction Stress Test (CST)

- Intravenous oxytocin (OCT) or breast stimulation (BSST) to stimulate ≥3 uterine contractions of at least 40 seconds long in 10 minutes period.
- Interpretation:
  - Negative: Absence of late or significant variable decelerations.
  - Positive: Presence of late decelerations after ≥50% of contractions.
  - Equivocal (suspicious): Intermittent late or significant variables decelerations.
  - Unsatisfactory: <3 contractions in 10 minutes.
- Indications: Suspected fetal or placental compromise, decreased fetal movement or abnormal NST >28 weeks, borderline AFI, and intrauterine growth restriction.
- Contraindications: History of or current preterm labor, preterm premature rupture of membranes, previous uterine surgery, placenta or vasa previa, undiagnosed bleeding.

Biophysical Profile

- Two points for presence of each of reactive NST, fetal breathing, fetal movement, fetal tone, and adequate amniotic fluid index. Maximum score 10 points.
- Interpretation and management:
  - 8–10 points: Normal.
  - 6 points: Equivocal. Should repeat in 12–24 hours or consider delivery.
  - 0–4: Abnormal. Consider delivery.
  - Oligohydramnios always warrants further evaluation.
- Indications: Suspected fetal compromise, nonreactive NST, decreased fetal movement >28 weeks, maternal indications (hypertension, diabetes), multiple gestation, borderline AFI, intrauterine growth restriction (IUGR), and fetal anomalies.

- Optimal time for testing is 2 hours after meal when breathing most likely observed.
- Contraindications: None.

Doppler Velocimetry

- Measurement of fetal umbilical artery or middle cerebral artery velocimetry.
- Interpretation: High middle cerebral artery (MCA) flow or elevated ratio of MCA to umbilical artery S/D ratio may be a predictor for fetal compromise.
- Indications: Suspected intrauterine growth restriction (IUGR), oligohydramnios, and fetal anemia.
- Contraindications: None.

Vibroacoustic Stimulation Test (VAS)

- Device generating acoustic and vibratory signal.
- Interpretation: In third trimester, expect to see transient increase in heart rate within 10 seconds of stimulus. Effect usually lasts several minutes.
- Indications: Nonreactive fetal heart tracing.
- Contraindications: None.

▶ DRUGS (TERATOGENIC/RECREATIONAL)

Basic Principles

- Increased volume of distribution and renal clearance in pregnancy can result in decreased plasma levels of drugs compared to pre-pregnancy state.
- Most drugs traverse the placenta by simple diffusion. Transplacental transfer rapid for drugs that are:
    - Molecular size <1000 daltons
    - Lipid soluble
    - Not charged
    - Not protein bound

Factors influencing transplacental drug transfer are molecular size, lipid solubility, degree of ionization, and protein binding.

Teratogenicity

- <2% of congenital anomalies are caused by drugs and chemicals.
- Preimplantation period (from fertilization to implantation):
    - Referred to as "all or none" period.
    - Insult that damages many cells usually kills embryo, but if only few cells injured, embryo usually able to compensate with normal growth and development.
- Embryonic period (weeks 2–8 after conception):
    - Period of organogenesis most critical for structural malformations.
- Fetal period (>9 weeks after conception):
    - Maturation and functional development occurs, with brain development particularly susceptible.

Recreational Drugs

ALCOHOL

- Most common cause of mental retardation.
- Can result in fetal alcohol syndrome, intrauterine growth restriction, microcephaly, ocular abnormalities, joint abnormalities, cardiac defects, behavioral disturbances, and craniofacial anomalies.

- Safe threshold dose in pregnancy not established. Highest risk of having affected child is women who drink >6 cups a day or engage in binge drinking.

TOBACCO

- Well-established cause of fetal growth restriction and other morbidities (see Prenatal Care section).

COCAINE

- Shown to cause spontaneous abortion, prematurity, intrauterine growth restriction, microcephaly, cerebral infarction, urogenital anomalies, and neurobehavioral disturbances.

HEROIN

- Not been shown to increase congenital anomalies.
- Withdrawal symptoms in neonate common. May increase risk of sudden infant death syndrome.
- Reports of developmental delay and behavioral disturbances in these children.

METHADONE

- May cause lower birth weight and withdrawal symptoms (more severe than from heroin due to longer half-life).

PHENCYCLIDINE (PCP)

- May increase incidence of behavioral and developmental abnormalities.

MARIJUANA

- Not shown to cause teratogenicity, but may be associated with low birth weight.

OTHER

- Caffeine, amphetamines, methamphetamines, and lysergic acid diethylamide (LSD) not been shown to be teratogenic in humans.

Medications as Teratogens

ANTICONVULSANTS

- Phenytoin:
    - Fetal hydantoin syndrome occurs in 5–10% born to pregnant women treated with phenytoin.

Maternal alcohol consumption is the leading cause of mental retardation.

OBSTETRICS

- Anomalies include intrauterine growth restriction, microcephaly, craniofacial anomalies, cleft lip/palate, limb defects, nail or distal phalangeal hypoplasia, hernias, broad nasal bridge, epicanthal folds, hypertelorism, and mental deficiency.
- **Carbamazepine:**
    - Unclear teratogenic potential, some evidence of craniofacial defects, fingernail hypoplasia, and developmental delay.
- **Valproic acid:**
    - Associated with neural tube defects
    - Reports of cardiac malformations, limb defects, craniofacial anomalies
- **Phenobarbitol:**
    - Not known to be teratogenic in humans.

WARFARIN

- Exposure in embryological period increases risk of **warfarin embryopathy**:
    - Nail hypoplasia
    - CNS defects
    - Stippled vertebral
    - Femoral epiphyses
- Exposure in second and third trimester increases risk of:
    - Corpus collosum agenesis
    - Dandy-Walker malformation
    - Midline cerebellar atrophy
    - Microphthalmia
    - Optic atrophy, blindness
    - Developmental delay
    - Mental retardation

ACE INHIBITORS AND ANGIOTENSIN RECEPTOR BLOCKERS (ARBs)

- Exposure >12 weeks may lead to oligohydramnios, renal anomalies, renal failure, pulmonary hypoplasia, hypocalvaria, growth restriction, and death.

RETINOIDS

- Unclear whether high doses of **vitamin A** are teratogenic.
- **Isoretinoin** and **etretinate** can have teratogenic effects on cranium, face, heart, CNS, and thymus.
- Etretinate has a very long half-life and can cause teratogenic effects even if conception occurs after discontinuation.
- **Tretinoin** (topical acne treatment) not teratogenic.

HORMONES

- **Androgens** can cause masculinization of female external genitalia and abnormal male genital growth.
- Progestins can cause masculinization of female fetuses and is associated with small increase in heart defects.
- Estrogens not teratogenic.
- **Diethylstilbestrol (DES)** exposure increases risk of abnormalities of vagina and uterus of fetus, including excess cervical eversion, vaginal

adenosis, hypoplastic uterus, septa, "withered fallopian tubes," and clear cell adenoma of vagina and cervix (risk of 1/1000).

ANTINEOPLASTIC DRUGS

- **Cyclophosphamide** in early pregnancy associated with hypoplastic or missing digits, cleft palate, single coronary artery, imperforate anus, and fetal growth restriction with microcephaly.
- **Methotrexate/Aminopterin** can cause growth restriction, failure of calvarial ossification, craniosynostosis, small ears, micrognathia, limb abnormalities, and hypoplastic supraorbital ridges.

ANTIMICROBIALS

- **Tetracycline** associated with stained teeth and hypoplasia of enamel.
- **Aminoglycosides** associated with 1–2% risk of ototoxicity.
- **Streptomycin** associated with cranial nerve VIII damage if given for long periods.
- **Sulfanomides** associated with hyperbilirubinemia when used near term.
- **Quinolones** associated with arthropathy in dogs, so rarely used in pregnancy.
- **Griseofulvin** increases CNS and skeletal anomalies in animal studies, but no known teratogenicity in humans.

OTHER EXPOSURES

- **Methylmercury** can cause cerebral atrophy, seizures, spasticity, and mental retardation.
- **Ionizing radiation** (large amounts) can cause mental retardation, microcephaly, and skeletal anomalies.

▶ NORMAL LABOR

Uterus

- In late pregnancy, gap junctions develop between adjacent myometrial cells.
- Gap junctions facilitate synchronization of uterine contractions.

Cervix

- Mostly composed of collagen (woven in a triple helix), elastin, smooth muscle cells, and glycosaminoglycans.
- Influence of estrogen and possibly relaxin breaks down collagen and replaces glycosaminoglycans with hyaluronic acid, making the cervix soft and distensible.

Pelvic Types

- See Figure 2-4 and Table 2-11 for review of the four types of pelvises.
- Most women do not have a "pure" pelvic type and present with combination of pelvic characteristics.

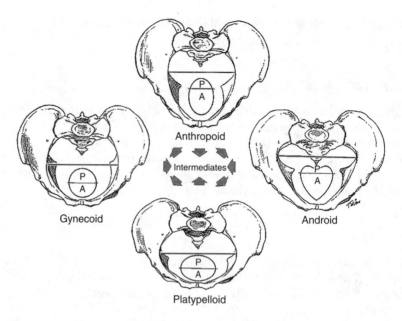

FIGURE 2–4. **Four pelvic types.**

(Reproduced, with permission, from Cunningham, et al. *Williams Obstetrics*, 21st ed. New York, NY: McGraw Hill, 2001:57, Fig 3-27.)

TABLE 2–11. **Pelvic Types and Characteristics**

PELVIC TYPE	GYNECOID	ANTHROPOID	ANDROID	PLATYPELLOID
Incidence	85%	7.3%	4.5%	3.1%
Shape	Round or ovoid	Ovoid with long AP diameter	Triangular, heart shaped	Transverse oval
Prognosis for vaginal birth	Good	Good	Poor	Poor
Inlet				
AP diameter	12.5 cm	Long	Adequate to short	Short
Transverse diameter	13.5 cm (adequate)	Adequate to narrow	Adequate	Wide
Midpelvis				
AP diameter	11.5 cm	Adequate	Short	Short
Transverse diameter	10.5 cm (adequate)	Adequate to short	Average	Wide
Outlet				
AP diameter	11.5 cm	Long	Short	Short
Transverse diameter	11 cm (adequate)	Adequate	Short	Wide

Mnemonic

"GAP"–describes pelvic shapes in order of their frequency:

Gynecoid
Android/anthropoid
Platypelloid

Initiation of Labor

- Placental hormones and uterine distension stimulate formation of myometrial gap junctions and oxytocin receptors.
- Fetal maturation results in prostaglandin production, which stimulates coordinated myometrial activity.

Normal Labor Progression

- **First stage** of labor consists of:
  - Latent phase: Slow effacement and dilation.
  - Active phase: Regular contractions and rapid rate of cervical change.
- **Second stage** is time from full cervical dilation to delivery.
- **Third stage** is time from delivery of infant to delivery of placenta.
- See Table 2-12 for a review of abnormal labor patterns.
- Predictors of abnormal labor progression are:
  - Narrow pelvic arch
  - Sharp or prominent ischial spines
  - Diagonal conjugate <11 cm
  - Fixed and forward inclining sacrum
  - Chorioamnionitis
- Progression of labor is the greatest predictor of pelvic adequacy.

The greatest predictor of pelvic adequacy is progress of labor.

TABLE 2-12. Labor Disorders and Therapies

STAGE	NULLIPAROUS	MULTIPAROUS	THERAPY
Prolonged latent phase	>20 hours	>14 hours	Therapeutic (pharmacological) rest or oxytocin
Protracted active phase	<1.2 cm/hour	<1.5 cm/hour	AROM, oxytocin (if inadequate contractions) Cesarean section (if adequate contractions)
Protracted second stage	<1 cm/hour	<2 cm/hour	Oxytocin (if inadequate contractions) Operative/assisted delivery (if adequate)
Arrest of dilation	No change in >2 hours	No change in >2 hours	AROM, oxytocin (if inadequate contractions) Cesarean section (if adequate contractions)
Arrest of descent	No change in >2 hours or >3 hours with epidural	No change in >1 hour or >2 hours with epidural	Oxytocin (if inadequate contractions) Operative/assisted delivery (if adequate)

TABLE 2-13. Bishop Scoring System

Factor	0	1	2	3
Cervical dilation	Closed	1–2	3–4	5+
Cervical effacement	0–30%	40–50%	60–70%	80+
Fetal station	–3	–2	–1	≥+1
Cervical consistency	Firm	Medium	Soft	
Cervical position	Posterior	Mid	Anterior	

Induction of Labor

- Elective induction of labor requires one of the following:
  - Fetal heart tones documented for 20 weeks by fetoscope or 30 weeks by doppler.
  - 36 weeks passed since positive serum or urine pregnancy test positive.
  - Ultrasound measurement of crown rump length at 6–12 weeks supports a gestational age ≥39 weeks.
  - Ultrasound at 13–20 weeks confirms gestational age of ≥39 weeks determined by clinical history and physical examination.
- The Bishop score is a predictor of the likelihood of a successful induction:
  - See Table 2-13 for Bishop scoring system.
  - Score ≤4 associated with up to 50% induction failure rate. Cervical ripening is indicated.
  - Score of >6 is favorable for successful induction.
  - See Table 2-14 for methods of cervical ripening.

TABLE 2-14. Agents for Cervical Ripening/Induction of Labor

Agent	Dose	Administration Schedule	Precautions	Oxytocin Initiation
PGE$_2$ gel (Prepidil) dinoprostone	2 mg	Every 6 hours, maximum three doses	Hyperstimulation (1%)	6 hours after last dose
PGE$_2$ insert (Cervidil) dinoprostone	10 mg sustained release	Place in posterior fornix for 12 hours	Hyperstimulation (5%) up to 9 hours after insertion	30–60 minutes after removal
PGE$_1$ tablet (Cytotec) misoprostol	25 µg	Every 4 hours	Should never be used in women with previous cesarean	4 hours after last dose
Intracervical Foley catheter	30 mL balloon	Insert above internal os for 12–24 hours	Shorter induction times, but no change in rate of cesarean	With placement or after removal

- ≥42 completed weeks from last menstrual period.
- Occurs in 10% of pregnancies.

Etiology and Risk Factors

- Error in dating (most common)
- Prior postdates pregnancy
- Primiparity
- Placental sulfatase deficiency (rare)
- Fetal anencephaly (rare)

Morbidity

- Increased risk of macrosomia, oligohydramnios, meconium, cesarean section, fetal heart decelerations, and abnormal labor pattern.
- Odds ratio for fetal death increases weekly after 41 weeks.
- Mortality rate increases significantly after 42 weeks.
- Between 41 and 42 weeks, assessment with one of these should be initiated:
  - Biophysical profile
  - Nonstress test with amniotic fluid index
  - Contraction stress test with amniotic fluid index

Management

- Delivery indicated if there is oligohydramnios, nonreassuring fetal assessment or if risk to fetus of continuing pregnancy is greater than induction of labor.

► VAGINAL BIRTH AFTER CESAREAN (VBAC)

Contraindications

- Women with any of the following should not be offered a trial of labor:
  - Previous classical or T-shaped uterine incision (rupture rate 4–9%)
  - Uterine surgery with entrance into endometrial cavity
  - Previous uterine rupture
  - Medical or obstetric complications precluding vaginal delivery
  - Inability to perform immediate cesarean (lack of continuous obstetric or anesthesia coverage)

Predictive Factors

- Overall success rates are 60–80%
- Factors associated with successful trial of labor are:
  - Prior vaginal delivery including previous VBAC
  - Low transverse uterine incision
  - Spontaneous onset of labor
  - Adequate pelvis
  - Previous cesarean done for a nonrecurring cause (e.g., breech presentation)
  - Maternal age ≤40

OBSTETRICS

Benefits of Trial of Labor

- Decreased risk of:
  - Thromboembolism
  - Wound infection
  - Febrile morbidity
  - Maternal discomfort
- Shorter hospital stay

Risks of Trial of Labor

- Maternal risks pertain to uterine rupture or need for cesarean delivery:
  - Uterine rupture (0.5–1% if low transverse incision)
  - Hemorrhage
  - Damage to adjacent organs
  - Anesthetic complications
  - Hysterectomy
- Fetal risks pertain to extrusion of fetus, cord, or placenta and include:
  - Hypoxia
  - Cerebral palsy
  - Mental retardation
  - Fetal or neonatal demise

Uterine Rupture

Most common sign seen with uterine rupture is fetal heart rate decelerations.

- No reliable predictors of uterine rupture.
- Risk increases with number of previous cesarean deliveries.
- Signs include:
  - Fetal distress (most common, seen in 70% of cases)
  - Pain
  - Loss of station
  - Vaginal bleeding
  - Bloody urine

▶ OPERATIVE DELIVERY

Operative Vaginal Delivery

- See Table 2-15 for a classification of operative vaginal deliveries.
- Indications for vacuum or forceps assisted delivery are:
  - Maternal exhaustion
  - Prolonged second stage of labor (>2 hours or >3 hours with epidural)
  - Fetal intolerance of labor
  - Prolonged moderate or severe variables
  - Maternal indications that contraindicate pushing
- The following are required prior to attempting assisted delivery:
  - Fetal head vertex and engaged
  - Position of fetal head precisely known
  - Cervix completely dilated
  - No cephalopelvic disproportion suspected
  - Empty maternal bladder
  - Adequate analgesia
- Complications are fetal scalp laceration, skull or nerve injury, retinal hemorrhage, elevated neonatal bilirubin, cervical laceration, fourth degree laceration, vaginal hematoma, postpartum hemorrhage, and urinary retention.

TABLE 2-15. Classification of Forceps and Vacuum Delivery

TYPE OF PROCEDURE	CLASSIFICATION
Outlet	Scalp visible at introitus without manually separating labia Sagital suture in anteroposterior diameter +/–45 degrees Rotation not to exceed 45 degrees (forceps)
Low	Leading point of fetal skull at or below +2 Sagital suture in anteroposterior diameter +/–45 degrees Any rotation over 45 degrees (forceps)
Mid	Above +2 station but engaged
High	Should not be performed

Cesarean Delivery

- Indications include prior cesarean delivery, arrest of dilation or descent, abnormal presentation, macrosomia (EFW >5000 g, or >4500 g if diabetic), non-reassuring fetal tracing, and prior uterine surgery.
- Complications are increased risk of endometritis, hemorrhage, thromboembolism, urinary tract infection, surgical injury to maternal organs, and death.

▶ EPISIOTOMY

Median

- Midline incision
- Advantages: Cosmetically superior, less pain
- Disadvantages: Increased incidence of third and fourth degree lacerations

Mediolateral

- Incision is 45–90 degree angle from midline.
- Advantage: Less damage to sphincter.
- Disadvantages: Greater blood loss, difficult to repair, more painful.

▶ OBSTETRIC ANESTHESIA

- Uterine contractions and cervical dilation cause visceral pain (T10-L1).
- Descent of fetal head and perineal stretching cause somatic pain by pudendal nerve (S2-4).

Parenteral (IV) Analgesia

- Opioid agonists or agonist-antagonists administered intermittently or by patient-controlled administration.
- Effect on pain relief is limited.

- Common agents are morphine, meperidine, fentanyl, nalbuphine, and butorphanol.
- Complications are neonatal sedation or respiratory depression, which can be reversed with *naloxone*.
- Should not be used if decreased variability or signs of fetal distress on fetal heart tracing.

Local Anesthesia

- Lidocaine (1%) often used prior to episiotomy or for laceration repair.
- Onset is rapid and can last 30–60 minutes.
- Adverse effects are uncommon and usually result from intravascular injection or excessive administration:
  - Central nervous system toxicity: Light-headed, dizziness, tinnitus, bizarre behavior, slurred speech, metallic taste, tongue or mouth numbness, muscle fasciculation, generalized convulsion, and loss of consciousness.
  - Cardiovascular toxicity: Hypertension and tachycardia, followed by hypotension, and cardiac arrhythmia.

Pudendal Block

- Transvaginal injection of lidocaine through sacrospinous ligament to pudendal nerve (S2-4).
- Complications are intravenous injection, hematoma formation (usually due to defective coagulation), and rarely infection.

Paracervical Block

- Injections at 3 and 9 o'clock positions of cervicovaginal junction.
- Can provide relief in first stage of labor.
- Transient fetal bradycardia reported in 10–70%, occurs within 10 minutes and lasts up to 30 minutes.

Spinal Anesthesia

- One time local infiltration of subarachnoid space with long-acting anesthetic.
- Provides pain relief for 30 minutes to 4 hours depending on medications used.
- Complications include:
  - **Hypotension** from sympathetic blockade. Treatment with intravenous fluids, ephedrine, and left lateral displacement of the uterus.
  - **Total spinal blockade** results in hypotension and apnea. Occurs promptly and may be followed by cardiac arrest if not quickly treated.
  - **Spinal headache** caused by CSF leak at injection site, which causes brain to shift caudad. Usually self-limited in 3–5 days. Improved by supine position, caffeine, hydration, or blood patch.
  - **Convulsions** rarely seen with cases of spinal headache.
  - **Bladder dysfunction** due to blunted sensation.
- Contraindications are coagulopathy, infection at insertion site, sepsis, uncorrected hypovolemia, increased intracranial pressure due to mass, recent use of low molecular weight heparin.

Epidural Anesthesia

- Local infiltration of potential space above dura given as single injection or repeated doses through an indwelling catheter.
- Complications include:
    - **Total spinal blockade** if dura inadvertently punctured.
    - **Ineffective analgesia**, failed or incomplete block occurs in 3–5%.
    - **Hypotension** from sympathetic blockade. Treatment is with intravenous (IV) fluids, ephedrine, and position change for left lateral displacement of uterus.
    - **Maternal fever** thought to be from imbalance between heat production and loss, altered hypothalamic thermoregulation or infection.
    - **Effect on labor** may include prolongation by 40–90 minutes. No statistical increase in operative delivery.
    - **Back pain** in 30–40% of patients after regional anesthesia.

General Anesthesia

- Indicated if there is:
    - Need for immediate cesarean delivery.
    - Contraindication to regional anesthesia.
    - Intraoperative failure of regional anesthesia.
    - Severe hemorrhage.
    - Need for uterine relaxation (head entrapment, uterine inversion).
- Complications include:
    - Failed intubation: 8% higher risk than nonpregnant patients.
    - Increased risk of aspiration.
    - Fetal CNS depression (anesthetic agents cross placenta).

▶ NEONATAL EVALUATION AND RESUSCITATION

Apgar Scores

- See Table 2-16 for a review of Apgar scoring.
- Used to evaluate status and need for resuscitation of newborn.
- Five observations given scores at 1 and 5 minutes and later if needed (usually until score of 7 reached).
- Scores of 7–10 are normal, 4–6 are intermediate, and 0–3 are low.
- Change between 1- and 5- minute scores is indicative of effect of resuscitation efforts. Not a good predictor of long-term neurological outcome.

TABLE 2-16.   Apgar Scoring System

	0	1	2
Heart rate	Absent	<100	>100
Respiratory effort	Absent	Weak cry, irregular	Good, strong cry
Muscle tone	Flaccid, limp	Some flexion	Active motion
Reflex irritability	No response	Grimace	Vigorous cry
Color	Blue or pale	Body pink, extremities blue	Completely pink

Resuscitation

- Algorithm for resuscitation found in Figure 2-5.
- Should always prevent heat loss by drying newborn and providing warm environment.
- Subsequent steps include clearing and suctioning airway and assessing breathing pattern, heart rate, and color.
- An infant with spontaneous respirations and a heart rate of >100 bpm does not require resuscitation.

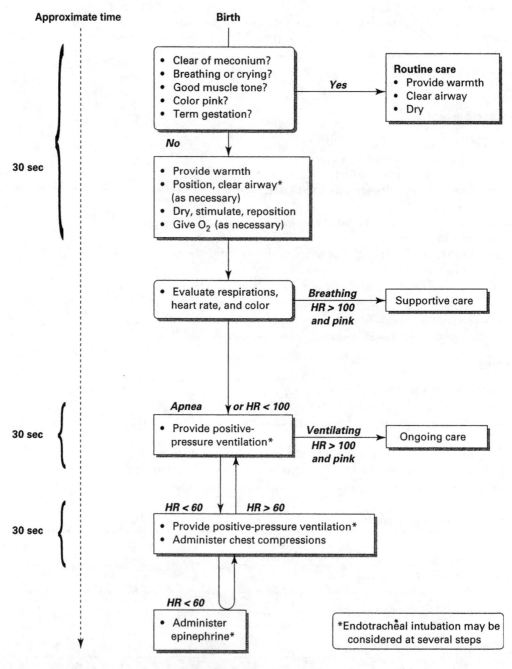

FIGURE 2-5. **Algorithm for resuscitation of the newborn.**

(Reproduced with permission from *Textbook of Neonatal Resuscitation*, 1987, 1990, 2001. Copyright © American Heart Association; DeCherney et al. *Current Obstetric & Gynecologic Diagnosis & Treatment*, 9th ed. New York, NY: McGraw-Hill, 2003:554, Fig. 29-1.)

Umbilical Cord Blood Gases and pH

- Normal umbilical cord blood gas values are seen in Table 2-17.
- Cord specimens kept at room temperature for up to 60 minutes show little change in pH and CO_2
- **Metabolic acidemia** develops when oxygen deprivation results in anaerobic metabolism which secretes lactic and β-hydroxybutyric acid.
- **Respiratory acidemia** results from CO_2 retention after acute disruption of placental gas exchange.
- **Base excess** is amount of remaining buffering capacity of bicarbonate. As metabolic acidemia occurs, bicarbonate concentration decreases and results in less base excess or more base deficit (expressed as negative base excess).
- Table 2-18 shows expected blood gas values with acidemia.

Eye Infection Prophylaxis

- To prevent neonatal gonococcal ophthalmia, the CDC recommends administration of erythromycin ointment, silver nitrate solution, or tetracycline ointment to newborns (ideally within first hour after birth).
- None of these treatments shown to provide effective prophylaxis for *Chlamydia* infection, so any infant with conjunctivitis <30 days of birth should be considered for chlamydial conjunctivitis.

Infant Circumcision

- American College of Obstetricians and Gynecologists (ACOG) and American Academy of Pediatrics (AAP) agree that there is insufficient evidence to recommend routine neonatal circumcision.
- Circumcisions often performed for religious, cultural, and prophylactic reasons, with rates varying from 40–80% of infants.
- Potential benefits:
  - Decreased rate of urinary tract infections (although overall risk is low)
  - Decreased rate of phimosis (although overall risk is low)
  - Possible decreased rate of sexually transmitted diseases and penile cancer

TABLE 2-17. Normal Umbilical Cord Blood Gas Values in Term Newborns

	ARTERIAL	VENOUS
pH	7.28 ± 0.15	7.34 ± 0.15
pO_2 (mmHg)	15 ± 10	30 ± 15
pCO_2 (mmHg)	45 ± 15	40 ± 8
Base excess (mEq/L)	-7 ± 4	-5 ± 4

TABLE 2-18. Umbilical Cord Blood Gas Values with Acidemia

	RESPIRATORY ACIDEMIA	METABOLIC ACIDEMIA	MIXED RESPIRATORY-METABOLIC ACIDEMIA
pH	↓	↓	↓
pO_2 (mmHg)	Normal	↓	↓
pCO_2 (mmHg)	↑	Normal	↑
Base excess (mEq/L)	Normal	↓ (more negative)	↓ (more negative)

- Risks and complications:
  - Bleeding (0.1%)
  - Infection
  - Injury to glans penis or urethra
  - Phimosis
- Analgesia should be given and options include EMLA, dorsal penile nerve block, and subcutaneous ring block.

▶ THE PUERPERIUM

The puerperium is the 6-week period after delivery during which the physiological and anatomic changes of pregnancy return to prepregnancy state.

Uterine Changes

- Uterine weight at term is 1000 g and decreases to 500 g within 2 weeks.
- By 4–6 weeks, uterus returns to normal size and is <100 g. The total number of cells does not change, but each cell decreases in size.
- Within 2–3 days after delivery, the decidua differentiates into superficial and basal layers. The superficial layer sloughs off (lochia) and basal layer gives rise to the new endometrial layer. Endometrium is fully restored by day 16.
- Lochia is composed of decidua, erythrocytes, bacteria, and epithelial cells.
- Placental site is ~9 cm after delivery and completely involuted by 6 weeks.
- Polymorphonuclear leukocytes persist in endometrium for 10 days. Plasma cells and lymphocytes may last for several months.

Cervical Changes

- 3 days after delivery, cervix appears normal but can be dilated up to 3 cm.
- Vascular hypertrophy and hyperplasia resolve by 6 weeks.
- Round cell infiltration and stromal edema can last up to 4 months.

Ovulation and Menstruation

- In non lactating women, the average time to ovulation (and return of menstrual cycle) is 7–9 weeks, with a range of 4–10 weeks.
- In lactating women, the average time to ovulation is 6 months with a range of 4 weeks to 9 months.

- Return of ovulation depends on frequency and proportion of formula supplementation. In exclusively breastfeeding women, 1–5% ovulate in first 6 months.
- Elevated prolactin released during suckling thought to be basis of ovulation suppression.
- FSH levels are the same in lactating and non-lactating women postpartum. Estrogen secretion suppressed in lactating women.

Lactation

- Milk secretion initially stimulated by fall in progesterone levels while prolactin remains high.
- Continued milk production dependent on nipple stimulation which induces oxytocin release from posterior pituitary.
- Colostrum, secreted postpartum days 2–5, contains:
  - More minerals and protein, less sugar and fat than mature milk.
  - Antibodies, such as immunoglobulin A, which provide some protection against enteric infections.
  - Macrophages, lymphocytes, and complement.
- Breastfeeding **contraindicated** in patients with:
  - HIV infection
  - HTLV-1 infection
  - Active untreated tuberculosis
  - Infant with galactosemia
  - Breastfeeding permissible in patients with cytomegalovirus, hepatitis B or C
- Medications contraindicated during breastfeeding include:
  - Bromocriptine
  - Cocaine and PCP
  - Cyclophosphamide
  - Doxorubicin
  - Ergotamine
  - Lithium
  - Methotrexate
  - Radioactive iodine
- Benefits of breastfeeding to infants are decreased risk of:
  - Rotavirus infection
  - Otitis and respiratory infections
  - Allergic and atopic disease
  - Juvenile onset diabetes
  - Hospital admissions in first year of life
- Bottle feeding more common in women with unwanted pregnancies and those who are young, not college educated, and of low socioeconomic status.
- Hormonal suppression of lactation (i.e., bromocriptine) not routinely indicated as it has been associated with seizures, myocardial infarctions, strokes, and psychiatric problems in postpartum women.

Urinary Tract Changes

- Epidural anesthesia and labor can temporarily decrease bladder function.
- Overdistention and residual urine occurs as bladder can have increased capacity and insensitivity to pressure.
- Early catheterization of patients with difficulty voiding helps prevent long-term urinary problems.

■ By 2–6 weeks postpartum, dilated ureters and renal pelvises return to normal size.

Cardiovascular System

■ Blood volume and cardiac output usually remain elevated 2–3 days postpartum from shift of extracellular fluid into vascular space and increased venous return.
■ Increased heart rate seen in pregnancy decreases within 2 days.
■ Blood volume, cardiac output, and heart rate usually return to normal by 2–6 weeks postpartum.

Hematological

■ Leukocytosis up to 30,000/uL, commonly seen intrapartum and postpartum.
■ Elevated fibrinogen and sedimentation rate seen during pregnancy remain elevated 1 week postpartum.

Immunizations

■ Patients who are Rh D-negative with Rh D-positive infants should receive anti-D immune globulin (RhoGAM) prior to discharge.
■ Rubella immunization (if not immune) and hepatitis B immunization (if at risk for infection) should be given prior to discharge. The vaccinations are not contraindications to breastfeeding.

Contraception

■ Contraception not necessary for first 3 weeks because of delay in ovulation.
■ In non-lactating women, contraception can be started after 2–3 weeks. Increased risk of thrombosis should be considered prior to initiation of combination oral contraceptives.
■ In lactating patients, nonhormonal methods should be considered first.
■ Hormonal contraceptives known not to affect quality of breast milk (progestin pills and depot medroxyprogesterone) usually initiated 3–6 weeks postpartum.
■ Impact of oral contraceptives with ethinyl estradiol is controversial and usually not recommended until ≥6 weeks after delivery in lactating women.
■ Lactational amenorrhea is effective form of contraception (98% in first 6 months) if patients breast-feed eight times per day with no supplementation and maximum intervals of 6 hours between feeding.

▶ POSTPARTUM COMPLICATIONS

Endometritis

Endometritis occurring after cesarean delivery is usually polymicrobial.

■ Most common cause of postpartum fever.
■ Frequency of infection 5–10 times greater after cesarean delivery, especially if women have had labor, rupture of membranes, or chorioamnionitis prior to cesarean section.
■ Endometritis after vaginal delivery usually caused by one type of bacteria.
■ Endometritis after cesarean delivery usually polymicrobial with aerobic (*Escherichia coli*, group B streptococci) and anaerobic (*Bacteroides*) bacteria.
■ Gold standard of treatment is gentamicin and clindamycin (curative in 85–95%), but alternatives include ampicillin-sulbactam, cefoxitin, ceftriaxone and metronidazole or levofloxacin and metronidazole.

Urinary Tract Infection

- Urinary tract infections, occurring in 5% of women, are second leading cause of postpartum fever.
- Predisposed by prolonged labor, urinary retention, and indwelling catheters.

Endometritis and urinary infections are the two most common causes of postpartum fever

Mastitis

- Risk factors are nipple trauma, engorgement, missed feedings, and plugged ducts.
- Common organisms are *Staphylococcus aureus*, *Streptococcus* species, and *Escherichia coli*.
- Treatment is dicloxacillin or cephalosporin for 10–14 days.
- Breastfeeding or pumping should be continued.
- Persistent fever may signify an abcess, which requires incision and drainage.

Wound Infection and Dehiscence

- Risk factors for wound complications are obesity, diabetes, smoking, cancer, malnutrition, cardiovascular disease, immunosuppressive therapy, and previous surgery.
- Approximately 2–15% of patients develop a wound infection after cesarean section. Rate is higher if cesarean delivery done after labor or with chorioamnionitis.
- Prophylactic (at time of cord clamp) antibiotic therapy been shown to decrease rate of wound infection after cesarean section.
- Epithelialization occurs within 48 hours after surgery, but epithelial layer is thin and easily traumatized.
- 60–80% of tensile strength obtained at 6 weeks after cesarean.
- Fascial dehiscence occurs in <1% of patients, usually occurs within 2 weeks with an average of 8 days postoperatively.
- Hematomas are more common than seromas and are usually the result of poor hemostasis.
- Small hematomas and seromas can be expectantly managed but large ones should be drained.
- Subcutaneous closure decreases incidence of wound seroma and separation in patients with wound thickness of ≥2 cm.

Episiotomy Infection and Dehiscence

- Infection of episiotomy is rare:
    - Has significant morbidity especially when associated with third or fourth degree laceration.
    - Diagnosis based on purulent discharge, erythema, and induration.
    - Treatment involves opening site, removing all sutures, copious irrigation, and debridement as well as treating with broad spectrum antibiotics.
- Dehiscence occurs in 0.1–2% of episiotomies and repair is:
    - Usually successful if done within 1–2 weeks.
    - Requires debridement of necrotic tissue and old sutures, daily irrigation, antibiotics if infection present, and oral bowel preparation night prior to repair.
    - Done similarly to primary closure.
    - Low residue diet and sitz baths recommended after repair.

Postoperative Ileus

- Ileus after cesarean delivery is uncommon.
- Symptoms include nausea, vomiting, absence of flatus, and abdominal distention.
- Treatment is with conservative measures including intravenous fluid administration, electrolyte replacement, and withholding oral intake.

Thromboembolism

- Thromboembolism (pulmonary embolism and deep venous thrombosis) is second most common cause of maternal death, second only to hemorrhage.
- Pregnancy increases the risk of thromboembolic events 5–50 folds.
- The risk of events is twofold greater after cesarean compared to vaginal delivery.

Amniotic Fluid Embolism

- The incidence of amniotic fluid embolism is reported to be 1 in 8000 to 1 in 80,000 deliveries.
- The mortality rate is ~60%, with rates reported to be 26–90%.
- Symptoms are nonspecific and include nausea, vomiting, agitation, dyspnea, and rapidly developing severe hypoxemia, cardiogenic shock, hypotension, disseminated intravascular coagulation, and hemorrhage.
- Fetal distress almost always present.
- Management is supportive with inotropic and vasoactive agents and fluid management.
- Survivors frequently affected with neurological sequela.
- More common in male fetuses and thought to be systemic inflammatory response to fetal tissue.
- Usually occurs intrapartum or immediately postpartum but can occur after first and second trimester abortions or after amniocentesis.

Postpartum Blues and Depression

POSTPARTUM BLUES

- Occurs in 30–80%.
- Rapid mood changes, including sad, irritable, anxious, tearful, and decreased concentration.
- Symptoms usually peak at 5 days and subside within 2 weeks.
- No conclusive data on etiology.
- Risk factors are personal or family history of depression, history of premenstrual mood disorder, and psychosocial impairment in work or personal relationships.
- Treatment is supportive.

POSTPARTUM DEPRESSION

- Occurs in 10%.
- Symptoms are loss of appetite, energy level, sleep, and libido.
- Timing of onset variable.

Postpartum blues occurs in 30–80% and postpartum depression occurs in 10% of women postpartum.

- Risk factors are postpartum blues, personal or family history of psychiatric illness, marital conflict, perceived lack of support, unplanned pregnancy, unemployment, stressful life events within previous year, and child care–related issues.

POSTPARTUM PSYCHOSIS

- Occurs in 1/1000.
- Medical emergency.
- Symptoms of depression, mania, schizoaffective, suicidal, or infanticidal thoughts.
- Risk factors are personal history of bipolar disorder (20–50% relapse rates), history of postpartum psychosis (70% relapse rate), or a family history of postpartum psychosis.

OBSTETRICS

CHAPTER 3

Complications of Pregnancy

Jeannine Rahimian, MD, MBA
Daniel A. Kahn, MD, PhD
Malini Anand, MD
Mor Tzadik, MD, MS
Caroline M. Colin, MD, MS

Classification

- Diabetes often classified into types:
    - Type 1: Insulin dependent, juvenile onset
    - Type 2: Noninsulin dependent, adult onset
    - Gestational: Diabetes beginning or first recognized in pregnancy
- White's Class classification of diabetes in pregnancy is outlined in Table 3-1. White's Class A1 and Class A2 are gestational.

GESTATIONAL DIABETES

SCREENING AND DIAGNOSIS

- All pregnant women screened unless meets all low-risk criteria (see Table 3-2).
- If high risk, screen at first visit, otherwise at 24–28 weeks gestation.
- **Screening Test**: 50 g 1-hour glucose challenge test:
    - Threshold 130 mg/dL: Sensitivity 90%, higher false positive rate
    - Threshold 140 mg/dL: Sensitivity 80%, lower false positive rate
- **Diagnostic Test**: 100 g 3-hour glucose tolerance test:
    - Performed if 1-hour screening test is positive.
    - Positive test is when two of four values are elevated.
    - Threshold for fasting, 1 hour, 2 hours, 3 hours in mg/dL:
        - 95/180/155/140 (Carpenter/Coustan)
        - 105/190/165/145 (National Diabetes Group)

RISKS TO PREGNANCY

- Increased risk of hypertensive disorder.
- Increased risk of macrosomia, hyperbilirubinemia, operative delivery, shoulder dystocia, and birth trauma.

TABLE 3-1. **White's Class of Diabetes in Pregnancy**

WHITE'S CLASS	AGE OF ONSET (YEARS)	DURATION (YEARS)	DESCRIPTION
A	n/a	n/a	Gestational diabetes: A1: Diet controlled A2: Medication requiring (insulin, glyburide)
B	≥20 or	<10	No vascular disease
C	10–19 or	10–19	No vascular disease
D	<10 or	≥20	Retinopathy or hypertension
F			Nephropathy (>500 mg/day proteinuria)
H			Arteriosclerotic heart disease
R			Proliferative retinopathy or vitreous hemorrhage
T			History of renal transplant

TABLE 3-2. **Low-Risk Criteria for Glucose Screening**

▪ Age <25 years
▪ BMI <25
▪ Not of high-risk ethnic group
▪ No previous history of abnormal glucose tolerance
▪ No history of diabetes associated adverse obstetric outcome
▪ No family history of DM

ANTEPARTUM MANAGEMENT

- Glycemic control:
    - Accuchecks done fasting and 1 or 2 hours postprandial
    - Diet: 30 kcal/kg/day
    - Start medication if fasting levels >95, 1 hour >140 or 2 hours >120:
        - Insulin is traditional therapy.
        - Glyburide is safe and efficacious in studies.
- Antepartum testing:
    - Twice weekly NST/AFI
    - Start at 28–34 weeks if poorly controlled, insulin requiring, or other risk factors
    - Start at 40 weeks if diet controlled
- Delivery:
    - If class A2 or B, generally induce around 39 weeks. May reduce incidence of macrosomia or shoulder dystocia but no evidence in controlled studies.

POSTPARTUM

- Lifetime risk of diabetes mellitus as high as 50%.
- Screening should be done at 6 weeks postpartum with fasting glucose or 2-hour glucose tolerance test.

PREGESTATIONAL DIABETES

RISK TO PREGNANCY

- Fetal:
    - Macrosomia
    - Intrauterine growth restriction
    - Spontaneous abortion
    - Congenital anomalies:
        - Four- to eightfold increase
        - CNS and cardiovascular most common
    - Respiratory distress syndrome due to delayed lung maturity
- Maternal:
    - Preterm birth
    - Hypertension or preeclampsia (class D, F, R at higher risk)

- Diabetic ketoacidosis:
  - Hyperglycemia results in osmotic diuresis, profound vascular volume depletion, and electrolyte depletion.
  - Signs are hyperventilation, obtunded mental state, dehydration, abdominal pain, and vomiting.
  - Diagnosis with blood sugar >200 mg/dL, serum HCO_3^- <18 mg/dL, metabolic acidemia, and serum ketones.
  - Treatment with volume resuscitation, insulin, and electrolyte repletion.

ANTEPARTUM MANAGEMENT

- Establish White's Class: 24-hour urine protein, serumcreatimine, ECG, and ophthalmological examination
- Serial ultrasounds to monitor growth
- Fetal echocardiogram at 20–22 weeks
- Glycemic control same as for gestational diabetes (see Gestational Diabetes section).
- Antepartum testing starting 28–34 weeks depending on risk factors and control
- Delivery:
  - Poor glucose control: Perform amniocentesis and induction at 37 weeks
  - Good glucose control: Induction around 39–40 weeks generally recommended
  - Offer cesarean section if estimated fetal weight >4500 g

INTRAPARTUM MANAGEMENT

- Keep glucose between 80 and 110 mg/dL to minimize risk of perinatal asphyxia or neonatal hypoglycemia.
- If good control: Avoid dextrose in intravenous (IV) solution.
- If poor control: Use dextrose IV with continuous insulin infusion to maintain euglycemia.

▶ RENAL DISEASE

Renal Function Assessment

- Urinalysis interpretation unchanged with pregnancy.
- Protein excretion may be increased, but proteinuria >300 mg/day is abnormal.
- Creatinine persistently >0.9 mg/dL is abnormal.
- Renal biopsy safe in pregnancy, but can usually be postponed.

Common Renal Diseases in Pregnancy

NEPHROLITHIASIS

- Calcium salts make up 80% of renal stones.
- Personal and family history increase risk of occurrence.

SYMPTOMS

- Flank pain and hematuria.
- May present with pyelonephritis resistant to antibiotic therapy.

DIAGNOSIS

- Urinalysis may show microscopic hematuria.
- Renal ultrasound sensitivity 85%.
- X-ray or one-shot IV pyelography useful if clinically suspicious with negative ultrasound.

TREATMENT

- IV hydration.
- Pain relief with narcotic analgesics if needed.
- Antibiotics if concomitant infection.
- Majority (75%) pass spontaneously. Ureteral stenting, percutaneous nephrostomy, lithotripsy, or basket extraction may be considered if necessary.

EFFECTS ON PREGNANCY

- No known adverse effects on pregnancy outcome
- Increased frequency of urinary infections

GLOMERULONEPHRITIS

SYMPTOMS

- Hematuria, proteinuria, renal insufficiency, edema, hypertension

DIAGNOSIS

- Renal biopsy shows membranous glomerulonephritis, IgA glomerulonephritis, or diffuse mesangial glomerulonephritis.

EFFECTS ON PREGNANCY

- Maternal hypertension develops in 50%.
- High risk of fetal loss, preterm delivery, fetal growth restriction.
- Risk of preterm delivery and growth restriction correlate to creatinine level.
- End stage renal failure may occur due to rapidly progressive glomerulonephritis or chronic glomerulonephritis.

NEPHROTIC SYNDROME

- Defect in glomerular capillary that allows excessive filtration of plasma proteins.
- Caused by primary glomerular disease, or immunological, toxic, or vascular injury.

DIAGNOSIS

- Proteinuria >3 g/day
- Hypoalbuminemia, hyperlipidemia, and edema

TREATMENT

- Increased dietary protein

EFFECTS ON PREGNANCY

- Presence of renal insufficiency or hypertension results in poor fetal and maternal outcome.

PREVIOUS RENAL TRANSPLANT

CHANGES AND SURVEILLANCE

- Glomerular filtration rate increases throughout pregnancy.
- Kidney dilates minimally to moderately.
- Should be closely monitored for hypertension and preeclampsia.
- Graft rejection is rare, but should be aggressively managed.

EFFECTS ON PREGNANCY

- Proteinuria develops in 40% cases, but usually not of significant level.
- Increased rate of preeclampsia, urinary infection, preterm delivery, premature rupture of membranes, and fetal growth restriction.

PREPREGNANCY EVALUATION

- Prior to attempting pregnancy, patients with history of a renal transplant should:
  - Not have severe hypertension for ≥2 years after transplant.
  - Have renal function stable without insufficiency, graft rejection, or proteinuria.

► INFECTIOUS DISEASES IN PREGNANCY

VARICELLA

- Infection tends to be more severe in adults and pregnant women than childhood.

SIGNS AND SYMPTOMS

- Rash
- Fever
- Respiratory distress in patients with pneumonia

DIAGNOSIS

- Based on clinical findings, recent exposure, and history.
- Varicella IgM may be sent for confirmation.

PREVENTION

- Varicella-Zoster immunoglobulin given within 96 hours of exposure prevents or minimizes infection.
- Vaccination in nonpregnant state if no history of varicella infection.

FETAL EFFECTS

- Infection <20 weeks can cause chorioretinitis, cerebral cortical atrophy, hydronephrosis, and cutaneous and bony leg defects.
- Infection >20 weeks associated with congenital varicella lesions and zoster.

MATERNAL EFFECTS

- Maternal mortality can be high if pneumonia is not treated.

COMPLICATIONS OF PREGNANCY

PARVOVIRUS

- Causes erythema infectiosum or **fifth disease**

SIGNS AND SYMPTOMS

- **Slapped cheek** appearance of bright red macular rash and erythroderma.
- Arthralgia may be present.
- Majority of women are asymptomatic.

DIAGNOSIS

- Presence of parvovirus specific IgM antibody

FETAL EFFECTS

- Can result in fetal death, miscarriage, hydrops, severe fetal anemia, or congenital abnormalities.

RUBELLA (GERMAN MEASLES)

SIGNS AND SYMPTOMS

- Low grade fever, headache, conjunctivitis, rash, arthralgia
- Subclinical in 25% of cases
- Viremia precedes rash by 1 week

DIAGNOSIS

- Presence of specific IgM antibody, peaks at 7–10 days after rash onset

PREVENTION

- Administration of rubella vaccine to susceptible women postpartum or preconception

FETAL EFFECTS

- Infection in first trimester more likely to cause congenital malformation than infection in second trimester.
- May result in miscarriage, stillbirth, or severe birth defects.
- **Congenital rubella syndrome:** Most common findings are cataracts, cardiovascular defects, sensorineural deafness, and mental retardation.

CYTOMEGALOVIRUS

- Most common cause of perinatal infection.
- Transmitted by droplet infection, contact with saliva and urine, through sexual contact, or reactivation of previous infection.

SIGNS AND SYMPTOMS

- Usually asymptomatic
- May have fever, pharyngitis, lymphadenopathy, polyarthritis

DIAGNOSIS

- Specific IgM antibody or fourfold increase in IgG antibody
- Recurrent infection not usually accompanied by IgM antibody
- CMV culture from amniotic fluid may be useful

PREVENTION

- No vaccine or screening method available

FETAL EFFECTS

- **Cytomegalic inclusion disease:** Low birth weight, microcephaly, intracranial calcifications, chorioretinitis, mental retardation, sensorineural deficits, hepatosplenomegaly, jaundice

TOXOPLASMOSIS

- Transmitted from raw or undercooked beef or pork, or through infected cat feces.
- One-third of adults in the United States have antibody to *Toxoplasmosis gondii*.

SIGNS AND SYMPTOMS

- Fatigue, muscle pain, lymphadenopathy
- Usually asymptomatic

DIAGNOSIS

- Specific IgM and IgG antibody.
- Ultrasound findings are microcephaly, ventriculomegaly, growth restriction, hydrops.
- Amniotic fluid tested by PCR.

PREVENTION

- Maternal immunity prior to pregnancy protects against fetal infection.

FETAL EFFECTS

- Classic triad is intracranial calcifications, chorioretinitis, and hydrocephalus.
- Other findings include low birth weight, hepatosplenomegaly, icterus, anemia, neurological disease, and mental retardation.
- Treatment with spiramycin or pyrimethamine plus sulfadiazine to women thought to be actively infected may reduce fetal infection.
- Frequency of infection greatest with infection in third trimester, but severity greatest with first trimester infection.

HERPES SIMPLEX VIRUS

- Herpes simplex virus (HSV)-1 causes oral herpes and 15–20% of genital herpes infections.
- HSV-2 causes majority of genital herpes infections.

SIGNS AND SYMPTOMS

- Painful vesicles on vulva, vagina, or cervix.
- Primary infection may include constitutional symptoms.

DIAGNOSIS

- Clinical examination.
- Specific IgM or IgG antibody.

- Culture of vesicle.
- Tzanck smear (cytological staining) is less sensitive than culture.

PREVENTION

- Prophylactic antiviral therapy reduces risk of recurrence and lesions during labor.
- Antiviral therapy should be started at 36 weeks if:
  - First episode during pregnancy
  - At risk for recurrence
- If lesions or distinct prodrome present, offer cesarean delivery.

FETAL EFFECTS

- Primary infection at time of vaginal delivery have high transmission rate (40%).
- Recurrent infection with overt lesion have small risk of transmission (5%).
- Asymptomatic shedding with no lesions has low risk of transmission (1%).
- Fetal infection may result in disseminated or localized lesions of central nervous system, eyes, skin, or mucosa.

GROUP B STREPTOCOCUS

- 10–30% of pregnant women colonized with group B streptococus (GBS) in vagina and/or rectum

SIGNS AND SYMPTOMS

- Usually asymptomatic

DIAGNOSIS

- Screening with culture of vagina and rectum at 35–37 weeks

PREVENTION

- Women who test positive for GBS should be treated with intrapartum antibiotics.
- If GBS status is unknown, should be treated by risk factors:
  - Previous infant with invasive GBS disease
  - Preterm labor (<37 weeks)
  - Membranes rupture ≥18 hours
  - Temperature ≥38°C
- Presence of GBS bacteriuria in any trimester should result in intrapartum treatment.

FETAL EFFECTS

- Early onset infection:
  - Occurs within 7 days of delivery
  - Incidence is 1–4 in 1000 live births
  - Signs of sepsis or severe pneumonia
  - Overall fatality 10–20%
- Late onset infection:
  - Occurs >7 days after delivery
  - Incidence 0.5–1.5 in 1000
  - Signs of pneumonia, bacteremia, meningitis

SYPHILIS

SIGNS AND SYMPTOMS

- Primary syphilis has appearance of chancre on vulva or cervix.
- Secondary syphilis may appear as rash or condyloma lata, usually 4–10 weeks later.
- May be asymptomatic.

DIAGNOSIS

- VDRL or RPR tests very sensitive but not specific
- FTA-ABS (fluorescent treponemal antibody absorption test) used for confirmation
- Amniotic fluid PCR for *Treponema pallidum*

PREVENTION

- All pregnant women should be screened at first prenatal visit and at delivery.
- Those who test positive should be tested for HIV.

FETAL EFFECTS

- May result in stillbirth, hydrops, edema, ascites, hepatosplenomegaly, skin lesions, lymphadenopathy, rhinitis, myocarditis.
- Highest rate of infection with primary or secondary syphilis. Lowest rate with late latent disease.
- Treatment is with penicillin. Antibiotic treatment can cause Jarisch-Herxheimer reaction, which may include uterine contractions and fetal distress.

GONORRHEA

SIGNS AND SYMPTOMS

- Dysuria, abnormal vaginal discharge.
- May be asymptomatic.
- Disseminated bacteremia may lead to skin lesions, arthralgias, septic arthritis, endocarditis, and meningitis.

DIAGNOSIS

- Genital culture
- Direct fluorescent antibody (DFA)
- PCR for DNA detection

PREVENTION

- Screening of all women at first prenatal visit.
- High-risk women should be screened again after 28 weeks.

FETAL EFFECTS

- Untreated gonococcal cervicitis associated with septic spontaneous abortion
- Increased risk of preterm delivery, premature rupture of membranes, chorioamnionitis, postpartum infection
- Treatment is with ceftriaxone or cefixime

CHLAMYDIA

SIGNS AND SYMPTOMS

- Often asymptomatic.
- Symptoms may include dysuria, abnormal vaginal discharge, conjunctivitis.

DIAGNOSIS

- DFA is more sensitive and specific than culture
- PCR for DNA detection

FETAL EFFECTS

- Neonatal conjunctivitis not prevented with eye prophylaxis given at birth
- Increased risk of neonatal pneumonia
- Controversial if increased risk of preterm delivery prematurely ruptured membranes

HUMAN IMMUNODEFICIENCY VIRUS

SIGNS AND SYMPTOMS

- Acute illness symptoms may include fever, night sweats, fatigue, rash, headache, lymphadenopathy, and pharyngitis.
- Opportunistic infections may be present in patients with AIDS.
- Often asymptomatic.

DIAGNOSIS

- Enzyme immunoassay (EIA) used for screening test with sensitivity of 99.5%
- Western blot or immunofluorescence used for confirmation

PREVENTION

- Screening of all pregnant women recommended at first prenatal visit.
- Treatment with zidovudine therapy reduces risk of transmission.
- Combination therapy with nucleoside analog and protease inhibitor very effective in suppressing RNA levels.
- Cesarean delivery recommended if viral load >1000 copies/mL.

FETAL EFFECTS

- Vertical transmission more common in preterm births, prolonged rupture of membranes, concomitant syphilis infection, and with breast-feeding.
- Increased risk of preterm delivery and low birth weight infant.
- Zidovudine can transiently lower hemoglobin of exposed infants.

HUMAN PAPILLOMAVIRUS

SIGNS AND SYMPTOMS

- Condylomata accuminata (genital warts) on vulva, vagina, or cervix
- Warts increase in number and size during pregnancy

PREVENTION

- Treatment of warts:
    - With trichloroacetic acid, cryotherapy, or laser therapy
    - In late second or third trimester to prevent presence during delivery
- Cesarean delivery only indicated if lesion large enough to prevent vaginal birth.

■ Laryngeal papillomatosis:
  ■ Transmission through aspiration at delivery
  ■ Caused by viral types 6 and 11

URINARY TRACT INFECTIONS

■ Majority of lower and upper urinary tract infections are caused by *Escherichia coli*, *Klebsiella pneumoniae*, and *Proteus* species.

SIGNS AND SYMPTOMS

■ Urinary frequency, dysuria, urgency.
■ Pyelonephritis symptoms also include fever, chills, flank pain.
■ Lower urinary infection may be asymptomatic.

DIAGNOSIS

■ Urinalysis with leukocytes and bacteria
■ Urine culture with:
  ■ ≥100 colonies and symptoms
  ■ ≥10,000 colonies and asymptomatic

PREVENTION

■ Screening culture should be done at first appointment for all obstetric patients.
■ Repeat urine culture should be done after treatment of infection to ensure cure.

FETAL EFFECTS

■ No teratogenic or malformations associated with urinary tract infections.

MATERNAL EFFECTS

■ Patients with pyelonephritis can develop:
  ■ Septic shock (1–2%)
  ■ Respiratory distress syndrome (1–2%)

TREATMENT

■ Lower tract infection: Oral antibiotic such as cephalosporin, nitrofurantoin, ampicillin, trimethoprim-sulfamethoxazole for 3–7 days.
■ Pyelonephritis: IV antibiotics until 24 hours afebrile, then oral antibiotics for 7–10 days.

BACTERIAL VAGINOSIS

SIGNS AND SYMPTOMS

■ Abnormal vaginal discharge with fishy odor, especially after intercourse

DIAGNOSIS

■ Clue cells on wet mount
■ Nitrazine positive (pH >4.5)
■ Positive whiff test (fishy odor after KOH administration)

FETAL EFFECTS

- Associated with premature rupture of membranes, preterm labor, chorioamnionitis, endometritis postcesarean delivery.
- Controversial whether treatment reduces risk of adverse outcomes.

▶ HEMATOLOGICAL DISORDERS

Anemia

- Definition during pregnancy difficult due to physiological changes and normal differences between individuals.
- Anemia usually refers to:
    - Hemoglobin <11 g/dL in first and third trimesters
    - Hemoglobin <10.5 g/dL in second trimester

IRON DEFICIENCY ANEMIA

CAUSES

- Associated with poor nutritional status.
- Occurs when iron requirements of pregnancy greater than amount absorbed through gastrointestinal tract.

DIAGNOSIS

- Microcytic anemia on complete blood count
- Serum ferritin levels low (<15 µg/L)
- % saturation (ratio of serum iron to iron-binding capacity) decreased

TREATMENT

- Iron therapy via ferrous sulfate or gluconate for total of 200 mg of elemental iron

EFFECTS ON FETUS

- Fetus usually not affected by iron deficient anemia of mother.

ANEMIA OF CHRONIC DISEASE

CAUSES

- Common diseases include chronic renal disease, inflammatory bowel disease, systemic lupus erythematosus, malignancy, and rheumatoid arthritis.

TREATMENT

- Often responds to erythropoietin administration

FOLIC ACID DEFICIENCY

CAUSES

- Inadequate consumption of folic acid, usually due to little consumption of green leafy vegetable, legumes, and animal protein.

DIAGNOSIS

- Low plasma folic acid concentration
- Macrocytic anemia
- Mean corpuscular volume elevated
- May develop nausea, vomiting, anorexia

TREATMENT

- Folic acid supplementation 1 mg/day

EFFECTS ON FETUS

- Fetus usually not affected by folate deficiency

SICKLE CELL DISEASE

CAUSES

- Most common sickle hemoglobinopathies are:
    - Sickle cell anemia (SS disease)
    - Sickle cell-hemoglobin C disease (SC disease)
    - Sickle cell-β-thalassemia disease (S-β-thalassemia disease)

DIAGNOSIS

- Hemoglobin electrophoresis analysis.
- Hemoglobin level usually doesn't fall below 7 g/dL.

TREATMENT

- Folic acid of 1 mg/day recommended because of increased folic acid requirements.
- IV hydration and oxygenation during labor, pain episodes, and anesthesia.
- Antepartum fetal surveillance at 32–34 weeks.
- Serial ultrasounds for fetal growth.
- Prophylactic red cell transfusion generally not recommended.

EFFECTS ON FETUS AND MOTHER

- Increased risk of perinatal mortality and spontaneous abortion
- Increased maternal morbidity, including:
    - Increased frequency of sickle cell crisis
    - Increased bacteriuria and pyelonephritis
    - Increased pneumonia, especially with *Streptococcus pneumoniae*
    - Risk of cardiac failure if hypertension or preeclampsia develops

β-THALASSEMIA MINOR

CAUSES

- Impaired production of β-globin chain causes excess α-chain and results in cell damage.

DIAGNOSIS

- Microcytic anemia and erythrocytes with stippling on peripheral smear.
- Iron levels usually normal or high.
- Hemoglobin electrophoresis shows high hemoglobin A_2 or F.

TREATMENT

- Recommendation of iron 60 mg and folic acid 1 mg

EFFECTS ON FETUS

- Both fetal and maternal outcomes unaffected

Thrombocytopenia

GESTATIONAL THROMBOCYTOPENIA

CAUSES

- Physiological decline in platelets

DIAGNOSIS

- Diagnosis of exclusion
- Will usually be >100,000/μL

TREATMENT

- Unnecessary to treat

EFFECTS ON FETUS

- No increased perinatal morbidity or mortality

IMMUNE THROMBOCYTOPENIC PURPURA

CAUSES

- Result of immune process with antiplatelet antibodies
- Mechanism of antibody production unknown

DIAGNOSIS

- Usually diagnosed prior to pregnancy

TREATMENT

- Treatment usually considered if count <50,000/μL.
- Corticosteroids may help increase platelet count.
- IV immunoglobulin may be given in refractory cases.
- Invasive techniques such as scalp electrode placement should be avoided.

EFFECTS ON FETUS

- Antiplatelet antibodies can cross placenta and cause neonatal thrombocytopenia.
- Increased risk of intracranial hemorrhage if severely thrombocytopenic (rare).

THROMBOTIC THROMBOCYTOPENIC PURPURA

CAUSES

- Microthrombi of hyaline material develop within arterioles and capillaries.
- Intravascular platelet aggregation leads to end-organ failure.

DIAGNOSIS

- Thrombocytopenia.
- Fragmentation hemolysis and hemolytic anemia.
- Variable organ dysfunction.
- Neurological symptoms (headache, altered consciousness, stroke) occur in 90% cases.

TREATMENT

- Plasmapheresis and exchange transfusion results in improved outcome
- Massive doses of glucocorticoid therapy

EFFECTS ON FETUS

- High perinatal morbidity and mortality

Deep Vein Thrombosis

CAUSES

- Stasis is single most predisposing factor.
- Thrombophilias (i.e., factor V Leiden mutation), cesarean delivery, and smoking are also risk factors.

DIAGNOSIS

- Symptoms include:
  - Abrupt onset severe pain and edema of leg and thigh
  - Pale, cool extremity with diminished pulsations
  - Calf pain
- Venography is gold standard, but Doppler ultrasound most often used for diagnosis.

TREATMENT

- Anticoagulation with therapeutic dose for 4 months, then low dose (see below)
- Bed rest until pain resolved, then gradual ambulation
- Analgesia

Anticoagulation in Pregnancy

- See Table 3-3 for indications and methods of anticoagulation in pregnancy.
- Treatment with unfractionated heparin or low-molecular weight heparin (LMWH).
- Decision on regimen and dose depends on indication for anticoagulation.

RISKS OF ANTICOAGULATION

- Heparin: Thrombocytopenia, bleeding, osteoporosis.
- LMWH: Cannot use in renal failure. May need dosage increase secondary to increased renal clearance and volume of distribution during pregnancy.

TABLE 3-3. Indication for and Methods of Anticoagulation in Pregnancy

	LOW DOSE PROPHYLAXIS		THERAPEUTIC DOSE	
Indications	■ Antiphospholipid syndrome ■ Thrombophilia carrier with personal or strong family history of thrombosis ■ History of idiopathic thrombosis		■ Artificial heart valve ■ Antithrombin III deficiency ■ Homozygous Factor V Leiden mutation ■ Homozygous prothrombin G20210A mutation ■ Antiphospholipid syndrome with history of thrombosis ■ History of life-threatening or recurrent thrombosis ■ Recent thrombosis	
Regimen	Heparin OR 5000–10,000 units SQ b.i.d.	LMWH Enoxaparin 40 mg q.d. Dalteparin 5000 units b.i.d.	Heparin OR ≥10,000 units SQ b.i.d. to t.i.d.	LMWH Enoxaparin 30–80 mg b.i.d. Dalteparin 5000–10,000 units b.i.d.
Monitoring	None needed	None needed	aPTT = 1.5–2.5 of normal	Peak (3 hours after dose) antifactor Xa levels q 4–6 weeks

PERIPARTUM MANAGEMENT WITH ANTICOAGULATION

- No regional anesthesia within 24 hours of last LMWH dose. Can consider switching to heparin SQ at 36–37 weeks gestation.
- High-risk patients (i.e., artificial heart valve, recent thrombosis) should receive heparin IV during labor and delivery. Others can have prophylaxis stopped at onset of labor.
- Anticoagulation should be restarted 4–8 hours after uncomplicated delivery as postpartum period is high risk.
- Anticoagulation should be continued for 6 weeks.

► CARDIOVASCULAR DISEASES

Diagnostic Evaluation

HISTORY AND PHYSICAL

- Cardiovascular disease can be difficult to diagnose during pregnancy as symptoms and clinical findings often similar to physiological changes in pregnancy.
- Cardiovascular disease should be suspected if:
  - Symptoms of orthopnea, nocturnal cough, hemoptysis, syncope, chest pain
  - Findings of cyanosis, clubbing, persistent neck vein distention, diastolic murmur, systolic murmur grade ≥3/6, cardiomegaly, persistent arrhythmia

DIAGNOSTIC STUDIES

ELECTROCARDIOGRAM

- Left-axis deviation of 15 degrees common due to diaphragm elevation.
- Mild ST-segment changes can be seen in inferior leads.
- Premature atrial and ventricular contractions are common.

Anticoagulation should be restarted 4–8 hours after an uncomplicated delivery as the postpartum period is very high risk.

- Tricuspid regurgitation and increased left atrial size are often normal findings in pregnancy.

CHEST X-RAY

- Heart silhouette often slightly enlarged in normal pregnancy, but gross cardiomegaly can be diagnosed with chest x-ray.

Common Cardiovascular Diseases

MITRAL STENOSIS

MATERNAL RISKS

- May result in significant pulmonary hypertension.
- Fixed cardiac output can result in ventricular failure and pulmonary edema due to increased preload of pregnancy.

MANAGEMENT

- Tachycardia often treated with beta blockers as decreased diastole time increases left atrial and pulmonary venous pressures.
- Limited physical activity recommended.
- Intrapartum care involves minimizing volume overload and endocarditis prophylaxis.

MITRAL INSUFFICIENCY

MATERNAL RISKS

- Generally well tolerated in pregnancy

MANAGEMENT

- Endocarditis antibiotic prophylaxis recommended

AORTIC STENOSIS

MATERNAL RISKS

- Mild-to-moderate stenosis well tolerated.
- Severe stenosis can result in fixed cardiac output.
- Decrease in preload decreases cardiac, cerebral, and uterine perfusion.

MANAGEMENT

- No treatment required for asymptomatic patient.
- If symptomatic, activity should be limited.
- Avoiding decreased preload and maintenance of cardiac output during labor is essential, therefore important to minimize hemorrhage and to be cautious with epidural.

AORTIC INSUFFICIENCY

MATERNAL RISKS

- Generally well tolerated in pregnancy

MANAGEMENT

- If symptomatic, should treat with bed rest, sodium restriction, and diuretics
- Endocarditis antibiotic prophylaxis recommended

ATRIAL SEPTAL DEFECT

MATERNAL RISKS

- Generally well tolerated in pregnancy
- Pulmonary hypertension is a rare complication

FETAL RISKS

- Risk of 5–10% of fetus being affected with an atrial septal defect

MANAGEMENT

- Treatment initiated if congestive heart failure or arrhythmia develops

VENTRICULAR SEPTAL DEFECT

MATERNAL RISKS

- If pulmonary artery pressure reaches systemic pressure level, right-to-left shunting occurs.
- Increased risk of pulmonary hypertension, Eisenmenger syndrome.

FETAL RISKS

- Risk of 5–10% of fetus being affected with a ventricular septal defect

MANAGEMENT

- Endocarditis antibiotic prophylaxis recommended if residual defect present.

PULMONARY HYPERTENSION

MATERNAL RISKS

- Mild-to-moderate hypertension well tolerated
- High maternal mortality in severe pulmonary hypertension

MANAGEMENT

- Limitation of activity, avoidance of supine position
- If symptomatic, treat with diuretics, oxygen, vasodilator agents
- Maternal mortality usually due to decreased venous return and right ventricular filling

MITRAL VALVE PROLAPSE

MATERNAL RISKS

- Generally well tolerated in pregnancy

MANAGEMENT

- If symptomatic, treat with beta-blockers to decrease sympathetic tone and palpitations
- Endocarditis antibiotic prophylaxis recommended if regurgitation or valvular damage

ASTHMA

SYMPTOMS AND DIAGNOSIS

- Wheezing, chest tightness, breathlessness.
- Severe exacerbations can result in hypoxemia, respiratory failure, death.

EFFECT OF PREGNANCY ON ASTHMA

- Symptoms worsen in 1/3 of patients
- Similar symptoms with each pregnancy

MATERNAL EFFECTS

- Increased incidence of preeclampsia, preterm labor, low birth weight infants, perinatal mortality.
- Status asthmaticus can result in maternal death.

FETAL EFFECTS

- Fetal hypoxemia can result from maternal alkalosis.
- Fetus can be affected before maternal oxygenation compromised.

MANAGEMENT

- Pulmonary function testing with peak expiratory flow rate (PEFR) or forced expiratory volume (FEV) most predictive.
- Inhaled corticosteroids and β-agonists are preferred treatment.
- Stress dose corticosteroids in labor if systemic steroids used within previous month.
- Ultrasound for fetal growth and antepartum testing based on severity of asthma.
- Prostaglandin $F_{2\alpha}$ (Hemabate) associated with bronchospasm and is contraindicated.

PULMONARY EMBOLISM

SYMPTOMS AND DIAGNOSIS

- Dyspnea, tachypnea, tachycardia, chest pain, cough, pleuritic pain, apprehension, hemoptysis.
- Ventilation-perfusion scan (VQ scan) shows perfusion defect and ventilation mismatch. Normal VQ scan can be seen with pulmonary embolism.
- Spiral computed tomography (spiral CT) also noninvasive, but less accurate for small emboli.
- Angiography is gold standard.

MANAGEMENT

- See Table 3-3 for anticoagulation during pregnancy.
- Bed rest and analgesia recommended until pain resolved.

- Anticoagulation with unfractionated or low-molecular weight heparin.
- Warfarin contraindicated during pregnancy, but recommended postpartum.

TUBERCULOSIS

SYMPTOMS AND DIAGNOSIS

- Cough, hemoptysis, night sweats
- PPD defined as positive if:
  - ≥ 15 mm in patient without risk factors ≥ 10 mm and foreign born, IV drug user, low-income population
  - ≥ 5 mm if HIV positive, abnormal chest x-ray, or recent contact

FETAL EFFECTS

- Congenital tuberculosis through placental infection is rare, but fatal

MANAGEMENT

- Treatment with isoniazid initiated during pregnancy if:
  - HIV positive
  - Recent exposure to active infection
  - Known recent converter
- If no risk factors, treatment delayed until postpartum and should be four drug treatment with isoniazid, pyridoxine, rifampin, ethambutol.
- Isoniazid toxicity includes hepatitis.

▶ GASTROINTESTINAL DISEASE

HYPEREMESIS GRAVIDARUM

SYMPTOMS AND DIAGNOSIS

- Severe nausea and vomiting unresponsive to therapy.
- Vomiting severe enough to cause weight loss, dehydration, acidosis from starvation.
- Mallory-Weiss tears and esophageal rupture is a rare complication.

TREATMENT

- IV fluid administration if dehydration severe
- Replacement of electrolyte deficits
- Antiemetic administration

REFLUX ESOPHAGITIS

SYMPTOMS

- Retrosternal burning due to relaxation of lower esophageal sphincter

TREATMENT

- Antacids
- Lifestyle changes (eating small meals, elevating head of bed)
- H_2-receptor antagonist or proton pump inhibitor

CHOLELITHIASIS

SYMPTOMS AND DIAGNOSIS

- Often asymptomatic
- Presence of gallstones on ultrasound of gallbladder
- Gallstone development increased with pregnancy

TREATMENT

- Prophylactic cholecystectomy unnecessary for asymptomatic stones
- Lithotripsy not recommended during pregnancy

CHOLECYSTITIS

SYMPTOMS AND DIAGNOSIS

- Right upper quadrant pain, anorexia, nausea, vomiting, low-grade fever, leukocytosis.
- Ultrasound shows gallstones.

TREATMENT

- Laparoscopic cholecystectomy is first-line treatment.

EFFECT ON PREGNANCY

- Occurrence during late gestation increases preterm labor.

PANCREATITIS

SYMPTOMS

- Epigastric pain, nausea, vomiting, abdominal distention
- Often have low-grade fever, tachycardia, hypotension
- Abdominal tenderness
- Serum amylase and lipase elevated
- Usually associated with cholelithiasis

TREATMENT

- Analgesics for pain
- IV hydration
- Prevent oral intake to decrease pancreatic secretion

HEPATITIS

SYMPTOMS AND DIAGNOSIS

- Nausea, vomiting, headache, malaise, low-grade fever.
- Jaundice usually develops 1–2 weeks after other symptoms.
- Elevated bilirubin, aminotransferase.
- Antibody positivity:
  - Hepatitis A: Hepatitis IgM antibody positive
  - Hepatitis B: Hepatitis B surface antigen (HBsAg) positive
  - Hepatitis C: Hepatitis C virus antibody positive

TREATMENT

- Supportive

EFFECTS ON PREGNANCY

- Minimal to no effect on pregnancy outcome
- Risk of hepatitis B transmission decreased with administration of hepatitis B immune globulin and vaccine to infant immediately after delivery
- No methods to prevent hepatitis C transmission

CHOLESTASIS

SYMPTOMS AND DIAGNOSIS

- Generalized pruritus is the most common symptom.
- May have icterus.
- Presence of cholic and chenodeoxycholic acid.

TREATMENT

- Ursodeoxycholic acid usually first-line treatment.
- Oral antihistamines provide symptomatic relief in some.
- Cholestyramine and dexamethasone have varying success.

EFFECTS ON PREGNANCY

- Increased rate of adverse outcome.
- More frequent abnormal fetal testing and meconium.
- Impaired vitamin K absorption can result in impaired coagulation.

ACUTE FATTY LIVER OF PREGNANCY

SYMPTOMS AND DIAGNOSIS

- Malaise, anorexia, nausea, vomiting, epigastric pain, progressive jaundice.
- Hypertension, proteinuria, and edema often confuse diagnosis with pre-eclampsia.
- Elevated bilirubin, low fibrinogen, prolonged clotting studies, elevated transaminases.
- Hypoglycemia is common.
- Hepatic coma, coagulopathy, and renal failure develop in about 50% cases.

TREATMENT

- Spontaneous resolution usually follows delivery.
- Treatment directed toward complications of sepsis, hemorrhage, renal failure, pancreatitis

EFFECTS ON PREGNANCY

- Hypovolemia and acidosis result in fetal mortality in 15–20% cases.

▶ NEUROLOGICAL DISEASES

Diagnosis of Neurological Diseases

- Most women with chronic neurological disease are diagnosed prior to pregnancy.
- New symptoms should be evaluated as in nonpregnant population.
- Cranial CT and MRI both safe in pregnancy.

SEIZURE DISORDER

IMPACT ON PREGNANCY

- Increased risk of congenital malformations due to epilepsy itself, anticonvulsant medications, or both.
- Congenital abnormalities seen in about 7% of infants.
- Some seizure disorders are inheritable, with 10% of children affected.

EFFECT OF PREGNANCY ON DISEASE

- Seizure frequency changes with pregnancy:
  - Increased in 35% women
  - Decreased in 15% women
  - No change in 50% women
- Increased frequency due to subtherapeutic medication levels, lower seizure threshold, or both.

HEADACHES

SYMPTOMS

- Tension headache characterized by:
  - Tightness with pain in back of neck
  - No neurological symptoms
  - Responds to massage, anti-inflammatory medications
- Migraine headache characterized by:
  - One-sided, throbbing pain
  - Nausea, vomiting often present
  - Aura or neurological symptom may be present

EFFECT OF PREGNANCY ON DISEASE

- Majority of women with migraine headaches have improvement with pregnancy.
- Some have onset of migraine headaches with pregnancy.

MYASTHENIA GRAVIS

SYMPTOMS

- Diplopia, ptosis common
- Easy fatigability of facial, extraocular, oropharyngeal, and limb muscles
- Course of disease variable

IMPACT ON PREGNANCY

- No effect on pregnancy outcome.
- Avoidance of magnesium sulfate, muscle relaxants, aminoglycosides.
- Higher rate of perinatal mortality.
- Transient symptomatic myasthenia gravis seen in infant due to transfer of embryonic acetylcholine receptors.

EFFECTS OF PREGNANCY ON DISEASE

- Does not affect course of disease
- Enlarging uterus may compromise respiration

MULTIPLE SCLEROSIS

SYMPTOMS

- Diplopia, loss of vision, weakness, hyperreflexia, spasticity
- Unpredictable, recurrent attacks of neurological dysfunction

IMPACT ON PREGNANCY

- No adverse effects on pregnancy outcome
- May have more fatigue.
- If bladder dysfunction present, have higher infection rate.

EFFECTS OF PREGNANCY ON DISEASE

- No adverse effects on disease course

▶ ENDOCRINE DISORDERS

Thyroid Disorders

HYPERTHRYOIDISM

SYMPTOMS AND DIAGNOSIS

- Tachycardia, thyromegaly, exophthalmos, heat intolerance
- Failure to gain weight despite normal or increased food intake
- Suppressed TSH level, elevated thyroxine (T_4) or triiodothyronine (T_3)

IMPACT ON PREGNANCY

- Outcome depends on metabolic control.
- Increased preeclampsia, abruption, preterm labor.
- Neonate may have transient thryotoxicosis or hypothyroidism.

EFFECT OF PREGNANCY ON DISEASE

- Increased incidence of heart failure if untreated due to combination of thyroxine and high output state of pregnancy.
- Pregnancy hormones may reduce severity of Graves disease.

MANAGEMENT

- Propylthiouracil (PTU).
- Methimazole less often used because:
  - More easily crosses placenta than PTU
  - Isolated reports of aplasia cutis
- Propranolol may be used for symptomatic relief.
- Thyroidectomy may be necessary if unable to treat medically. Increased vascularity due to pregnancy may cause increase in complication rate.

HYPOTHYROIDISM

SYMPTOMS AND DIAGNOSIS

- Usually diagnosed prior to pregnancy.
- Fatigue, feeling cold, constipation, loss of hair
- Low free thyroxine and high thyrotropin levels

IMPACT ON PREGNANCY

- Increased incidence of preeclampsia, abruption, low birth weight infant, stillbirth.
- May cause abnormal mental development if untreated.

EFFECT OF PREGNANCY ON DISEASE

- Increased incidence of heart failure

MANAGEMENT

- Thyroxine therapy
- Thyrotropin levels measured every 4–6 weeks with goal to be at lower level of normal

Adrenal Disorders

PHEOCHROMOCYTOMA

SYMPTOMS AND DIAGNOSIS

- Paroxysmal attacks of hypertension, headaches, profuse sweating, palpitation, apprehension
- Often manifest as hypertensive crisis, seizure disorder, anxiety attack.
- May also have chest pain, nausea, vomiting, pallor, flushing
- 24-hour urine vanillylmandelic acid (VMA), metanephrines, or unconjugated catecholamines is diagnostic

IMPACT ON PREGNANCY

- Complications associated with hypertension

EFFECT OF PREGNANCY ON DISEASE

- Increased incidence of maternal death

MANAGEMENT

- Hypertension management with α-adrenergic blocker
- Surgical exploration and tumor removal if necessary

CUSHING SYNDROME

SYMPTOMS AND DIAGNOSIS

- Moon facies, buffalo hump, truncal obesity
- Fatigability, weakness, hypertension, hirsutism, cutaneous striae, easy bruising
- Elevated plasma cortisol, not suppressible with dexamethasone

IMPACT ON PREGNANCY

- Increased incidence of preterm delivery and perinatal mortality

EFFECT OF PREGNANCY ON DISEASE

- Increased incidence of hypertension, gestational diabetes, heart failure

MANAGEMENT

- Treatment of hypertension.
- Transsphenoidal resection of pituitary adenoma or removal of adrenal adenoma can be done during pregnancy, if necessary.

Pituitary Disorders

PROLACTINOMA

See Chapter 5 (Reproductive Endocrinology and Infertility [REI]) under hyperprolactinemia section.

Parathyroid Disorders

HYPERPARATHYROIDISM

SYMPTOMS AND DIAGNOSIS

- Usually minimal symptoms, including fatigue, depression, confusion, anorexia, hyperemesis, constipation, nephrolithiasis, peptic ulcer disease.
- Hypercalcemic crisis includes stupor, nausea, vomiting, weakness, fatigue, dehydration.

IMPACT ON PREGNANCY

- Increased preterm delivery and stillbirth
- Hypocalcemia with or without tetany in infant

EFFECT OF PREGNANCY ON DISEASE

- Improvement of symptoms as renal excretion increased and calcium shunted to fetus.

MANAGEMENT

- Surgical removal of parathyroid adenoma is preferred management.
- Oral phosphate therapy is an option to postpone parathyroidectomy until after delivery.
- Hypercalcemic crisis treated with IV hydration and furosemide.

► COLLAGEN VASCULAR DISORDERS

Systemic Lupus Erythematosus

PATHOPHYSIOLOGY

- Tissues and cells damaged by autoantibodies and immune complexes
- Unknown etiology, but genetic influences likely
- Increased risk of disease if HLA-DR2 or HLA-DR3 genes present

SIGNS AND SYMPTOMS

- Malaise, fever, arthritis, rash, pleuropericarditis, photosensitivity, anemia, cognitive dysfunction
- Renal involvement common

DIAGNOSIS

- Antinuclear antibody (ANA) good for screening, but not very specific
- Anemia, thrombocytopenia, leukopenia
- Diagnosis requires presence of criteria from different organ systems

MATERNAL EFFECTS

- Outcome is better if:
  - Minimal disease activity ≥6 months prior to pregnancy
  - No active renal involvement
  - No development of superimposed preeclampsia
  - No antiphospholipid antibody activity
- Hypertension and proteinuria commonly develop or worsen
- Preexisting nephropathy is a risk factor for preeclampsia development

FETAL EFFECTS

- Presence of anti-SS-A and anti-SS-B increases risk of fetal cardiac dysfunction (congenital heart block) and dermatological manifestations.
- Increased perinatal morbidity and mortality due to vasculopathy, placental infarction, and decreased perfusion.
- Neonatal lupus erythematosus involves skin lesions, cardiac, or hematological abnormalities.

MANAGEMENT

- Frequent hematological, renal, and hepatic evaluation
- Fetal growth monitoring for growth restriction
- Nonsteroidal anti-inflammatory drugs for arthralgias
- Low dose aspirin if indicated for antiphospholipid syndrome
- Corticosteroids, immunosuppressive, cytotoxic agents for active disease

Antiphospholipid Antibody Syndrome

PATHOPHYSIOLOGY

- Antiphospholipid antibody (LAC) or anticardiolipin antibody (ACL) are prothrombotic antibodies.
- Phospholipid binding proteins such as protein C and protein S may also be involved in syndrome.

SIGNS AND SYMPTOMS

- Antiphospholipid antibody syndrome:
  - Recurrent arterial or venous thrombosis, thrombocytopenia, and fetal loss
  - 5–12% risk of thrombosis during pregnancy and postpartum
  - Present in 35% of women with lupus
- Prolonged coagulation studies (PT, PTT)

DIAGNOSIS

- Indications for testing of antibodies can be found in Table 3-4.
- Must satisfy ≥1 clinical criteria and ≥1 lab criteria
- Clinical criteria:
  - Arterial or venous thrombosis
  - ≥1 unexplained death of normal fetus after 10 weeks

TABLE 3-4. Indications for Testing for Antiphospholipid Antibodies

■ Recurrent pregnancy loss
■ Unexplained second or third trimester pregnancy loss
■ Arterial or venous thrombosis
■ Unexplained intrauterine growth restriction
■ Early onset severe preeclampsia
■ False positive syphilis serology test (RPR)

- ≥1 premature birth of morphologically normal neonate ≤34 weeks due to preeclampsia or severe placental insufficiency
- ≥3 unexplained spontaneous consecutive losses ≤10 weeks gestation
- Lab criteria must be positive on two occasions >6 weeks apart:
  - Anticardiolipin antibody (IgG, medium to high positive)
  - Lupus anticoagulant

MATERNAL EFFECTS

- Arterial and venous thrombosis
- Preeclampsia, often early onset
- Thrombocytopenia
- Neurological disorders
- Dilated postpartum cardiomyopathy

FETAL EFFECTS

- Fetal death, especially in second or third trimester
- Placental infarction
- Intrauterine growth restriction
- Libman-Sacks endocarditis

MANAGEMENT

- Treatment indicated if:
  - Presence of lupus anticoagulant and a previous pregnancy loss, or
  - High titer anticardiolipin antibody
- Treatment aimed at counteracting action of antibodies and includes:
  - Low dose aspirin (60–80 mg/day) blocks conversion of arachidonic acid to thromboxane A
  - Heparin (5000 to 10,000 units subcutaneous every 12 hours) to prevent thrombotic events
  - Immunoglobulin if heparin contraindicated or if first-line options failed

Rheumatoid Arthritis

PATHOPHYSIOLOGY

- Cause unknown
- T cells secrete cytokines that mediate inflammation
- Genetic predisposition and association with HLA-DR4

SIGNS AND SYMPTOMS

- Chronic polyarthritis
- Inflammatory synovitis usually involving peripheral joints
- Fatigue, anorexia, weakness, weight loss commonly seen
- May also have rheumatoid nodules, vasculitis, pulmonary symptoms

EFFECTS OF PREGNANCY

- Pregnancy has a protective effect for disease onset and decrease in symptoms.

FETAL EFFECTS

- No adverse outcome

MANAGEMENT

- Pain relief with:
  - Acetaminophen
  - Nonsteroidal anti-inflammatory agents
  - Aspirin
- Glucocorticoid agents (prednisone) if needed
- Hydroxychloroquine, sulfasalazine, gold salts, cyclosporine used with caution

PSYCHIATRIC DISORDERS

Mental Status Examination

- Tests cognitive function with specific questions on:
  - Orientation—year, date, season, location
  - Recognition—ask name of objects
  - Attention and calculation—serial 7s, spelling "world" backwards, following three-step command

Common Disorders

BIPOLAR DISORDER

SYMPTOMS

- Manic episodes alternating with depressive episodes
- Often have impaired social functioning

RISK IN PREGNANCY

- Symptoms may result in noncompliance with prenatal care.
- Delusions or hallucinations may result in harm to patient or fetus.

TREATMENT

- Usual treatment is with antidepressants or lithium

SCHIZOPHRENIA

SYMPTOMS

- Delusions, hallucinations, incoherence, inappropriate affect
- Deterioration of work and social functioning over time
- Onset of illness often around age 20

TREATMENT

- Antipsychotic agents include dopamine antagonists and clozapine

DEPRESSION

SYMPTOMS

- Weight loss or gain, loss of energy, sleep disturbances

RISK IN PREGNANCY

- Incidence is highest in second trimester and postpartum
- Increased risk for postpartum depression and psychosis
- May result in noncompliance with prenatal care, poor weight gain, suicidal ideation, impaired bonding with infant

TREATMENT

- Selective serotonin reuptake inhibitors (SSRIs) are primary line of treatment.
- Tricyclic antidepressants, serotonin norepinephrine reuptake inhibitor (SNRI) can be continued if symptoms well controlled rather than changing medication during pregnancy.

OBSESSIVE COMPULSIVE DISORDER

SYMPTOMS

- Uncontrollable urge to carry out particular behavior or rituals.
- Persistent, unwanted thoughts that cause anxiety or distress.
- Obsessions or compulsions are time consuming and cause distress or interfere with social functioning.

RISK IN PREGNANCY

- Obsession may be to harm the baby
- Rarely may lead to psychosis
- Usually worsens in postpartum

TREATMENT

- Pharmacological treatment, usually SSRIs, only in severe cases

EATING DISORDERS

SYMPTOMS

- Below normal body weight
- Lack of weight gain over multiple visits

RISK IN PREGNANCY

- Symptoms often improve as patients will eat to care for fetus.
- Weight gain can cause severe psychological distress.

TREATMENT

- Dietary habits should be monitored closely.
- Pharmacological treatment considered only in severe cases.

Medication Risks and Benefits

- Almost all psychotropic medications cross placenta, so risk of treatment must be weighed with risk of mood disorder.
- SSRIs and SNRIs are preferred because of good safety profile and adequate data.
- Usually best not to change medication during pregnancy if patient at risk for relapse or inadequate control with new medication.

SSRIs

- Includes fluoxetine, paroxetine, sertraline
- Most data on SSRIs compared to other antidepressant or antipsychotic medication
- No increased risk of anatomical malformations, miscarriage, prematurity
- Third trimester SSRI use associated with neonatal behavioral syndrome, with symptoms such as mild tremors, mild tachypnea, or seizures

SNRIs

- Includes venlafaxine
- No increased risk of anatomical malformations or miscarriage

TCA

- No increased risk of anatomical malformations or miscarriage in retrospective studies
- Desipramine and nortriptyline preferred because less sedative, less side effects

MONOAMINE OXIDASE INHIBITORS (MAOIs)

- Not recommended in pregnancy because of possible increased intrauterine growth restriction and lack of data

▶ SECOND TRIMESTER LOSS

SYMPTOMS AND CLINICAL MANIFESTATION

- Vaginal bleeding
- Vaginal or pelvic pressure
- Uterine contractions
- Dilation of cervix
- Low back pain
- Leakage of fluid
- Hour glassing of membranes through cervical os
- Fevers, purulent, or foul smelling discharge if infectious

CAUSES OF SECOND TRIMESTER LOSS

- Infection accounts for up to 40%
- Genetic or chromosomal account for 30–40%
- Uterine anomalies accounts for up to 25–30%.

- Antiphospholipid antibody syndrome accounts for 20%
- Cervical incompetence accounts for 10%
- Hypothyroidism is uncommon

INFECTIOUS CAUSES

- See page 54 (Infection diseases in Pregnancy)

GENETIC OR CHROMOSOMAL CAUSES

- See Chapter 2 (Obstetrics)

SEPTATE UTERUS

- Most common uterine abnormality associated with recurrent pregnancy loss
- Miscarriage rate >60%
- The longer the septum, the worse the prognosis
- Mechanism is poorly understood. May be due to poor blood supply or poor implantation

ANTIPHOSPHOLIPID ANTIBODY SYNDROME

- See antiphospholipid antibody section on page 76.

CERVICAL INCOMPETENCE

- Inability of uterine cervix to retain pregnancy in absence of contractions or labor.
- Most patients have no risk factors. Risk factors include:
  - Initial cervical length <22 mm has 10 times increased risk of preterm birth
  - In utero diethylstilbestrol (DES) exposure: 25–50% have structural abnormalities
  - History of trauma such as cervical laceration, prolonged second stage of labor, cervical dilators, treatment of cervical neoplasia
  - Uterine overdistention due to multiple gestation or polyhydramnios
- Diagnostic criteria:
  - Repetitive painless second trimester losses without contractions or bleeding
  - Significant premature cervical effacement or dilation (>2 cm)
  - Sonographic findings:
    - Cervical length ≤2.5 cm
    - Funneling of membranes into endocervical canal

HYPOTHYROIDISM

- High rate of first trimester abortion associated with untreated hypothyroidism, also contributes to second trimester losses.

DIAGNOSIS

- Thorough physical exam
- Ultrasound to evaluate signs of uterine anomaly

- Laboratory tests for infection, antiphospholipid antibody syndrome, thyroid disease, thrombophilias.
- Amniocentesis. Values consistent with infection are:
  - Glucose <14.
  - LDH >400.
  - Gram stain or culture positive.
- Genetic analysis of products to test for chromosomal abnormalities.

MANAGEMENT

- If bleeding but has normal cervical length and positive cardiac activity:
  - Continue close follow-up for resolution versus spontaneous miscarriage.
  - Counsel on increased risk of preterm delivery, fetal death, and perinatal death.
- If consistent with cervical incompetence: Consider emergency cerclage
- If infection present:
  - Expedite or induce delivery
  - Treat with broad spectrum antibiotics
- If fetal demise: Medical induction or surgical curettage

RECURRENCE AND PREVENTION

- Recurrence rate depends on cause of pregnancy loss.
- Antiphospholipid syndrome: Increased risk of loss with next pregnancy can be reduced with treatment such as heparin or aspirin.
- Cervical incompetence: Preventive cervical cerclage may decrease risk of future loss, but this is controversial.
- Uterine anomaly: Most common associated with fetal loss are bicornuate, septate, and didelphic. Consider resection of the septum if recurrent pregnancy loss.
- Infection: Most common are chlamydia, mycoplasma, and bacterial vaginosis organisms. Should treat when present, but screening of asymptomatic women not recommended.

▶ PRETERM LABOR

CAUSES OF PRETERM LABOR

- Infection which can be clinical or subclinical
- Placental abruption
- Psychological stress associated with preterm labor
- Uterine distention (i.e., multiple gestation)
- Often will not be able to identify cause for preterm labor or birth

RISK FACTORS

- Previous preterm birth
- Second trimester bleeding
- Polyhydramnios
- Risk of incompetent cervix (i.e., uterine anomalies, previous cone biopsy)
- Multiple gestation

DIAGNOSIS

- Definition is cervical dilation of ≥1 cm, effacement ≥80%.
- Ultrasound measurement of cervical length useful in predicting preterm birth.

- Fetal fibronectin has high negative predictive value, but poor positive predictive value. Should only be done if:
  - Amniotic membranes intact.
  - Cervical dilation <3 cm
  - Gestational age >24 and <34
- Amniocentesis can be done to assess for infection, but has not been shown to improve pregnancy or fetal outcome. Values of fluid consistent with infection are:
  - Gram stain positive bacteria (most specific)
  - Decreased glucose
  - Elevated white blood cell count
  - Elevated interleukin 6 count (most sensitive)

MANAGEMENT

- Treat infection (i.e., urinary, vaginitis) if present.
- Attempt to avoid delivery until ≥34 weeks with use of tocolytics such as:
  - Calcium channel blocker (nifedipine)—inconclusive data on whether delays delivery. Combination with magnesium sulfate increases risk of hypotension and cardiovascular collapse.
  - β-adrenergic agents (terbutaline)—delays delivery for no more than 48 hours. No proven benefit to outcome. Not FDA approved for preterm labor treatment.
  - Magnesium sulfate—studies show little difference in outcome.
  - Indomethacin—can be used <32 weeks.
- Antibiotic treatment (i.e., penicillin G) recommended if <37 weeks and group B *Streptococcus* status unknown.
- Corticosteroid administration with betamethasone or dexamethasone:
  - Decreases neonatal morbidity (respiratory distress, intraventricular hemorrhage) and mortality
  - Consider if risk of preterm delivery between 24 and 34 weeks
  - Consider if preterm rupture of membranes <32 weeks
  - Best if course completed >24 hours and <7 days before delivery
- Cerclage placement can be considered if incompetent cervix rather than preterm labor.
- Although bed rest commonly recommended, no evidence that it prevents preterm delivery.

▶ THIRD TRIMESTER BLEEDING

PLACENTAL ABRUPTION

- Premature separation of placenta from implantation site

RISK FACTORS

- Preeclampsia or hypertension
- Increased maternal age or parity
- Preterm rupture of membranes
- Cigarette smoking
- Cocaine use
- Trauma

DIAGNOSIS

- Usually associated with pain, contractions, or labor
- May or may not be visualized on ultrasound

- May lead to shock, coagulopathy, or fetal death if unrecognized
- Positive Kleihauer-Betke test is consistent with fetal to maternal hemorrhage and may be consistent with abruption

MANAGEMENT

- Delivery required
- Can await vaginal delivery if fetal status reassuring

RECURRENCE

- Risk of recurrence is 10 times greater, from 0.4 to 4%.

PLACENTA PREVIA

- Placenta located over or very near to internal cervical os:
    - Complete previa—placenta completely covers internal cervical os
    - Partial previa—placenta partially covers internal cervical os
    - Marginal previa—edge of placenta is at edge of internal cervical os
    - Low-lying placenta—placenta is in lower uterine segment but does not reach internal cervical os

RISK FACTORS

- Maternal age—increased in women ≤19 or ≥35
- Multiparity
- Previous cesarean section
- Cigarette smoking

DIAGNOSIS

- Classically painless vaginal bleeding
- Ultrasound provides confirmation, with transvaginal ultrasound superior to abdominal

MANAGEMENT

- Cervical examination should never be performed
- Vaginal delivery should not be attempted
- If hemorrhage is severe or if in labor, immediate delivery recommended
- Cesarean delivery should be planned at term
- Preterm fetus with no active bleeding should be observed closely

RECURRENCE

- Increased risk of recurrence

VASA PREVIA

- Fetal vessels course through membranes over cervical os
- Very uncommon
- High rate of fetal death
- Apt test will turn brown if blood is maternal and remain red if blood is fetal
- Emergency cesarean indicated regardless of gestational age if bleeding with vasa previa

Vaginal bleeding in presence of vasa previa is indication for immediate cesarean delivery.

LABOR

- Bloody show due to labor can present as third trimester bleeding. Other causes of bleeding, such as placental abruption, placenta previa, and vasa previa must be ruled out.

GENITAL TRACT ABNORMALITIES

- Abnormalities of the genital tract such as a cervical polyp, vaginal laceration from intercourse, or cervical cancer or dysplasia can result in third trimester bleeding.
- A thorough speculum exam should be performed to evaluate the vagina and cervix if other causes of bleeding excluded.

▶ HYPERTENSIVE DISORDERS

CAUSES OF HYPERTENSION

- See Table 3-5 for diagnostic criteria of hypertension in pregnancy
- Causes of hypertension include:
  - Gestational hypertension
  - Chronic hypertension
  - Preeclampsia (mild, severe, or superimposed)

TABLE 3-5. Diagnostic Criteria for Hypertensive Disorders in Pregnancy

DIAGNOSIS	CRITERIA
Gestational hypertension	■ BP >140/90 after 20 weeks ■ No proteinuria ■ BP normalizes within 12 weeks postpartum
Chronic hypertension	■ BP >140/90 prior to pregnancy or <20 weeks gestational age
Mild preeclampsia	■ BP >140/90 after 20 weeks ■ ≥300 mg protein on 24-hour urine collection
Severe preeclampsia	■ BP >160/110 after 20 weeks ■ ≥5 g protein on 24-hour urine collection ■ Symptoms (headache, visual disturbances, epigastric pain) ■ Laboratory abnormalities (e.g., creatinine >1.2, platelets <100,000)
Superimposed preeclampsia	■ Chronic hypertension without proteinuria <20 weeks ■ New onset of proteinuria >300 mg/24 hour ■ Blood pressures significantly increased above first trimester levels
Eclampsia	■ Seizure activity with hypertensive disorder

RISK FACTORS

- Nulliparity (2/3 of cases)
- Extremes of age
- Diabetes or obesity
- Personal or family history of preeclampsia or hypertension
- Multiple gestations

SIGNS AND SYMPTOMS

- See Table 3-5 for diagnostic criteria.
- Symptoms may include persistent headache, visual changes, epigastric pain.
- Signs may include hyperreflexia, pulmonary edema, petechiae, and generalized bruising.

LABORATORY TESTS

- Renal
  - Uric acid is most sensitive indicator of preeclampsia.
  - Creatinine.
  - Protein on 24-hour urine collection or 30 mg/dL (1+) on urinalysis.
- Hematological: Elevated hematocrit, thrombocytopenia, evidence of hemolysis
- Liver function tests: AST and ALT as indicator if microangiopathic anemia
- Coagulation studies abnormalities seen, often with consumptive coagulopathy in patient with severe preeclampsia

MATERNAL COMPLICATIONS

- See laboratory tests for discussion on hemolysis, coagulopathy, liver function
- Increased risk of:
  - Cerebrovascular accident
  - Seizure may occur antepartum, intrapartum, or postpartum
  - Renal failure from tubular necrosis, reduced perfusion, reduced GFR
  - Pulmonary edema due to decrease in plasma oncotic pressure
  - HELLP syndrome involves hemolysis, elevated liver enzymes, low platelets
  - Placental abruption

FETAL COMPLICATIONS

- Uteroplacental insufficiency
- Intrauterine growth restriction
- Preterm delivery

INDICATIONS FOR DELIVERY

- Mild preeclampsia ≥37 weeks
- Severe preeclampsia with signs of worsening disease
- Evidence of hepatic involvement, delivery recommended
- Worsening fetal status (intrauterine growth restriction or abnormal Doppler studies)

MANAGEMENT

ANTEPARTUM

- Efficacy of home bed rest compared to hospitalization is unclear.
- Expectant management of severe preeclampsia beyond 30 weeks controversial.
- Antepartum testing recommended starting 32–34 weeks.
- Treatment in chronic hypertension:
  - Reduces maternal risks of significantly elevated BP.
  - Beta-blockers may have some effect on fetal growth.
  - α-Methyldopa has good safety profile.
  - Diuretics increase perinatal mortality and blunt plasma volume expansion.
  - ACE inhibitors contraindicated due to fetal death in animal studies and renal agenesis in humans.

INTRAPARTUM

- Seizure prophylaxis:
  - Most seizures occur intrapartum and postpartum. No reliable predictors of seizure. Up to 24% have no proteinuria.
  - Magnesium is most effective agent in preventing seizures primarily through stabilization of membrane potentials.
  - Phenytoin not as effective as magnesium. Minimal fetal and maternal side effects. Recommended when magnesium contraindicated (myasthenia gravis, renal failure).
- Antihypertensive medication such as hydralazine, labetalol, or nifedipine recommended if systolic BP >160 or diastolic >105 mmHg.

RISK OF RECURRENCE

- Recurrence rate ranges from 5 to 45%.
- The earlier the gestational age at diagnosis, the higher the risk of recurrence.

▶ MULTIPLE GESTATIONS

RISK FACTORS

- Assisted reproductive technology
- Maternal age
- Increasing parity
- Family history of twins

DIAGNOSIS

- Uterine size greater than dates
- Ultrasound is confirmatory, with multiple gestational sacs seen after 5 weeks
- If fetuses are different genders or if two placentas seen, then dichorionic twins
- Chorionicity determined most accurately by examining membranes after delivery

MATERNAL RISKS

- Antepartum increased risk of:
  - Hypertension and preeclampsia increased with number of gestations
  - Placental abruption
  - Anemia
  - Urinary tract infection
  - Gestational diabetes
  - Abnormal placentation
- Intrapartum and postpartum increased risk of:
  - Operative delivery
  - Endometritis
  - Hemorrhage

FETAL RISKS

- Preterm delivery common. Mean gestation decreases as number of gestations increase.
- Perinatal mortality is threefold greater for twins than singletons.
- Increased risks of chromosomal abnormality independent of maternal age.

MANAGEMENT

- Fetal growth:
  - Serial ultrasounds for growth every 3–4 weeks or more frequent if discordant
  - Growth of twins comparable to singletons until 30–32 weeks
  - Discordant growth is a 20% difference in fetal weight
- Cervical length ≤2.5 cm at 24 weeks associated with increased risk of delivery <32 weeks, but shortened cervix at 28 weeks not predictive of preterm delivery.
- Fetal well-being should be monitored:
  - BPP useful if NST impractical because of number or position of fetuses.
  - Quantification of amniotic fluid volume not been firmly established. Methods that have been advocated:
    - Overall AFI (disregarding membrane)
    - Largest pocket in each sac
    - Subjective assessments
- Delivery can be vaginal for twins if both fetuses are vertex presentation. Cesarean recommended if presenting twin is breech or if more than two fetuses.

Complications of Multiple Gestations

TWIN-TWIN TRANSFUSION SYNDROME

- Occurs in 5–15% of monochorionic and rare dichorionic twin pregnancies.
- Exact cause unknown. Vascular anastomosis implicated but they occur in many monochorionic pregnancies not complicated by the syndrome.
- Donor twin: Anemia, oligohydramnios (maximum pocket <2 cm), stunted growth.
- Recipient twin: Plethoric polyhydramnios (maximum pocket >8 cm).
- Treatment is with serial amniotic fluid reductions, amniotic septostomy, and selective photocoagulation of communicating vessels.

Twin-twin transfusion syndrome occurs in 5–15% of monochorionic twin pregnancies.

MONOCHORIONIC-MONOAMNIONIC TWIN GESTATION

- 1% of monozygotic twins.
- Diagnosis made when membrane not seen on ultrasound, or entangled umbilical cords.
- High perinatal mortality rate due to:
    - Cord accidents
    - Prematurity
    - Growth restriction
    - Twin-twin transfusion syndrome
- Monitoring is controversial. Can hospitalize and monitor continuously until heart tracing nonreassuring or perform outpatient nonstress tests and admit when variable deceleration "significant" or more "frequent."
- Timing of delivery usually by 34 weeks.
- Mode of delivery is vaginal if possible, but cesarean frequently performed as there have been cases of transection of a nuchal cord that belonged to twin B.

INTRAUTERINE DEMISE OF ONE FETUS

- Vanishing twin or first trimester demise of one twin occurs in approximately 20% of twins diagnosed in first trimester. No prognostic effect on remaining pregnancy.
- Second or third trimester loss less common.
    - Significant risk for neurological complications (multicystic encephalomalacia) in surviving twin if monochorionic.
    - Immediate delivery may not protect surviving twin from neurological injury especially if premature.
- Maternal risk of disseminated intravascular coagulopathy (DIC) is low.

MULTIFETAL REDUCTION

- Reduction of triplets or quadruplets may be beneficial because of:
    - Increased length of gestation
    - Increased birth weights
    - Reduced prematurity and perinatal mortality
- Often offered if known chromosomal or structural abnormality

► INTRAUTERINE GROWTH RESTRICTION

RISK FACTORS

- Constitutionally small mother
- Poor maternal weight gain and nutrition
- Lower socioeconomic status (likely due to smoking, alcohol, drugs)
- Chronic renal disease
- Abnormal placentation
- Previous infant with growth restriction

DEFINITIONS

- Usually defined as estimated weight <10th percentile for gestational age.
- Increased morbidity and mortality inversely related to percentile (i.e., <3rd percentile has greater morbidity than <10th percentile).

- Asymmetric intrauterine growth restriction (IUGR) is disproportionately lagging abdominal growth.
- Symmetric IUGR proportionally small, often due to early insult such as chromosomal abnormality.
- Serial ultrasound measurements necessary to diagnose growth restriction.

CAUSES OF IUGR

- Infection—viral, toxoplasmosis, syphilis
- Toxin exposure—drugs, cigarette smoking, medications
- Congenital malformation or chromosomal abnormality
- Placental insufficiency—chronic hypertension, preeclampsia, antiphospholipid antibody syndrome
- Medical conditions—diabetes, chronic pulmonary or cardiac disease, hyperthyroidism
- Multiple gestation

MANAGEMENT

- Should evaluate for fetal anomalies
- Antepartum monitoring to assess fetal well-being with:
  - Nonstress test
  - Biophysical profile
  - Doppler velocimetry of umbilical artery
- No evidence that bed rest improves outcome
- Delivery at 37 weeks or earlier if documented fetal lung maturity

FETAL EFFECTS

- Increased risk of neonatal morbidity and mortality including:
  - Meconium aspiration
  - Hypoglycemia and hyperbilirubinemia
  - Seizures, sepsis, death
- Infants with growth restriction due to chromosomal or congenital viral factors generally remain small throughout life, whereas those due to placental insufficiency catch up after birth.

RECURRENCE RISK

- Risk of growth restriction increased in subsequent pregnancies.

Mnemonic for IUGR

Inherited: chromosomal, genetic
Uterine: placental insufficiency
General: maternal malnutrition, smoking
Rubella and other congenital infections

► MACROSOMIA

Definition

- Defined as fetal weight ≥4500 g

RISK FACTORS

- Maternal diabetes
- Obesity of parents
- Post-term pregnancy
- Maternal age or multiparity
- Male fetus
- Previous infant with weight >4000 g

DIAGNOSIS

- Usually not made until after delivery
- Ultrasound predictions often inaccurate

COMPLICATIONS

- Increased risk of:
  - Arrest of dilation or descent
  - Shoulder dystocia

MANAGEMENT

- Prophylactic labor induction not recommended
- Elective cesarean should be considered if:
  - Estimated weight ≥5000 or ≥4500 g in diabetic woman

▶ ISOIMMUNIZATION

- A mother lacking a specific red cell antigen can produce antibodies when exposed to fetal blood cells that have inherited the antigen from the father.
- Isoimmunization occurs rarely because of:
  - Insufficient transplacental passage of antigen or antibody
  - Variability of maternal immune response to antigen

Major Antigen Groups

- ABO blood group system:
  - About 20% have incompatibility and 5% are clinically affected.
  - Usually mild disease such as jaundice and anemia.
- Rhesus blood group system:
  - Includes five red cell proteins: c, C, D, e, E
  - Highest incidence is D negativity
- Other Blood groups:
  - Kell antigen uncommon, but results in severe fetal anemia and fetal death.
  - Kidd and Duffy can cause erythroblastosis, but tend to be mild.

Results of Incompatibility

- Immune hydrops:
  - Hemolysis can lead to cardiac enlargement, hepatic dysfunction, hydrops fetalis.
  - Severe anemia can result in intrauterine demise.
  - Live born infants appear pale, edematous, and limp. Dyspnea and circulatory collapse are common.

- Hyperbilirubinemia:
  - Marked hyperbilirubinemia can lead to kernicterus.
  - Anemia can persist for months.

- Only maternal red cell IgG antibodies are potentially harmful because IgM antibody cannot cross the placenta.
- Critical titer is titer equal to or higher that will cause severe hemolytic disease.
- Methods of determining fetal blood type:
  - Isolation of fetal cells from maternal serum
  - Amniocentesis
  - Chorionic villus sampling
  - Cordocentesis
- Antepartum testing for fetal well-being via:
  - Doppler studies of middle cerebral artery
  - Ultrasound assessment for immune hydrops
  - Amnionic fluid bilirubin concentration
    - Measured as ΔOD 450 and interpreted with Liley graph zones, which correspond to expected fetal anemia.
    - Transfusion indicated if value is zone 3 or rising zone 2.
  - Cordocentesis is intrauterine sampling of fetal blood for hemoglobin and reticulocyte count. Associated with higher risk than amniocentesis.

▶ PREMATURE RUPTURE OF MEMBRANES

Definition

- Rupture of the amniotic membranes before onset of labor
- If ≥37 weeks, premature rupture of membranes (PROM)
- If <37 weeks, preterm premature rupture of membranes (PPROM)

- Ascending infection causing cytokine cascade
- Physiological weakening associated with apoptosis and collagenase activity
- Placental abruption triggers thrombin
- Incompetent cervix
- May be unknown

- Sterile speculum exam.
  - Pooling test: Fluid collection visualized in posterior fornix.
  - Nitrazine test: Vaginal pH >6.0 or positive test is consistent with amniotic fluid. False positive with blood, semen, and bacterial vaginosis.
  - Ferning: Dried amniotic fluid becomes distinctive pattern resembling fern.
- Ultrasound will demonstrate reduced amniotic fluid volume.
- Indigo carmine dye injection via amniocentesis is absolute diagnosis when dye is visualized in the vagina.

MANAGEMENT

TERM (≥37 WEEKS)

- Expectant management if in labor.
- If not in labor, risk of induction weighed against risk of infection. About 90% will spontaneously go into labor within 24 hours of membrane rupture.
- Penicillin if GBS positive or if GBS status unknown with risk factors.

PRETERM (<37 WEEKS)

- Assess for infection with wet mount, GBS, gonorrhea, Chlamydia, and urine culture.
- If signs of chorioamnionitis, delivery recommended.
- If <32 weeks, administer corticosteroids, IV antibiotics, and attempt to prolong latency. About 50% with PPROM spontaneously go into labor within 24 hours of membrane rupture.
- Can test fetal lung maturity via vaginal pool or amniocentesis.
- Tocolytics are generally not recommended.

COMPLICATIONS

- Increased risk of chorioamnionitis with prolonged rupture of membranes
- Umbilical cord prolapse depending on cervical dilation and station
- Oligohydramnios may lead to:
    - Cord compression and variable decelerations
    - Pulmonary hypoplasia and Potter syndrome if <26 weeks gestation
- Placental abruption
- Fetal demise with PPROM depends on gestational age

▶ FETAL DEATH

CAUSES OF FETAL DEATH

FETAL CAUSES

- Chromosomal anomalies
- Birth defects
- Nonimmune hydrops
- Infection

PLACENTAL CAUSES

- Abruption
- Fetal-maternal hemorrhage
- Umbilical cord accident
- Placental insufficiency
- Placenta previa

MATERNAL CAUSES

- Antiphospholipid antibodies
- Diabetes

- Hypertensive disorders
- Trauma
- Sepsis, acidosis, or hypoxia
- Uterine rupture
- Post-term pregnancy

DIAGNOSIS

- Methods that can aid in determining cause of death include:
  - Autopsy
  - Chromosomal analysis especially if structural abnormalities noted
  - Viral serologies and bacterial cultures for infectious etiologies
  - Placental pathology
  - Kleihauer-Betke test can estimate volume of fetal blood in maternal circulation, which would be indicative of fetal to maternal hemorrhage

COMPLICATIONS

- Infection
- Hemorrhage
- Coagulopathy

▶ POSTPARTUM HEMORRHAGE

Definition

- Postpartum hemorrhage (PPH) is:
  - Estimated blood loss ≥500 mL after vaginal delivery, or
  - Estimated blood loss ≥1000 mL after cesarean section, or
  - Decrease in hematocrit of ≥10%
- Early PPH is ≤24 hours of delivery
- Late PPH is >24 hours and <6 weeks after delivery

CAUSES OF PPH

EARLY POSTPARTUM HEMORRHAGE

- Uterine atony most common. Risk factors include:
  - Uterine distention (multifetal gestation, polyhydramnios, macrosomia)
  - Protracted labor or prolonged use of oxytocin
  - Multiparity
  - Chorioamnionitis
  - Magnesium sulfate administration
- Retained placental fragments, placenta accreta
- Vaginal or cervical laceration
- Uterine inversion
- Uterine rupture
- Coagulopathy

LATE POSTPARTUM HEMORRHAGE

- Subinvolution of placental site
- Infection
- Retained products of conception

TABLE 3-6. Uterotonic Agents for Treatment of Postpartum Hemorrhage

MEDICATION	DOSE	FREQUENCY	CONTRAINDICATION	SIDE EFFECT
Oxytocin (pitocin)	10–40 units in 1 L of NS	Continuous infusion	None	Rare
Methylergonovine (Methergine)	0.2 mg IM	Every 2–4 hours	Hypertension, preeclampsia	Hypertension, nausea
15-Methyl-PGF$_{2\alpha}$ (Hemabate)	0.25 mg IM	Every 15–90 minutes. Max of 2 mg. (8 doses)	Asthma, renal, or hepatic disease	Gastrointestinal, flushing
Misoprostol	1000 µg /rectum	One dose	None	Gastrointestinal, headache

MANAGEMENT OF PPH

EARLY POSTPARTUM HEMORRHAGE

- Uterine massage.
- Uterotonic agents (see Table 3-6).
- Ultrasound can be used to:
  - Visualize retained placenta
  - Perform guided sharp curettage
- Uterine tamponade with packing.
- Uterine artery embolization.
- More invasive methods include uterine artery ligation (O'Leary stitch), internal iliac (hypogastric) artery ligation, and hysterectomy.

LATE POSTPARTUM HEMORRHAGE

- Treatment initially with uterotonics (Methergine, misoprostol, Hemabate).
- If infection suspected, treat with antibiotics.
- If uterotonic failed or retained products suspected, curettage should be performed.

▶ DERMATOLOGICAL DISORDERS IN PREGNANCY

PRURITIC URTICARIAL PAPULES AND PLAQUES OF PREGNANCY (PUPPPs)

SIGNS AND SYMPTOMS

- Erythematous lesions, with papules and plaques. Occasional vesicles, purpura
- Begins in abdominal striae with periumbilical sparing
- Spreads to thighs, buttocks, breasts, arms. Usually sparing face, palms, soles
- Average duration 6 weeks or until delivery

ETIOLOGY

- Unknown. May be inflammatory response triggered by rapid abdominal connective tissue distension.

PUPPPs begins in abdominal striae with periumbical sparing

TREATMENT

- Topical corticosteroids, antihistamines, or antipruritic medications.
- Severe cases may require a short course of oral corticosteroids.

FETAL EFFECTS

- No adverse effects

RECURRENCE

- Seldom recurs in subsequent pregnancy

PRURIGO OF PREGNANCY (PRURIGO GESTATIONIS)

SIGNS AND SYMPTOMS

- Erythematous papules and nodules on extensor surfaces of extremities. Sometimes on abdomen. Lesions may be crusted or excoriated.
- Persists through gestation and often into postpartum.

ETIOLOGY

- Unknown. May be related to atopic predispositon

TREATMENT

- Topical corticosteroids or antipruritic medication
- Oral corticosteroids if necessary

FETAL EFFECTS

- No adverse effects

RECURRENCE

- Variable recurrence in subsequent pregnancies

HERPES GESTATIONIS (PEMPHIGOID GESTATIONIS)

SIGNS AND SYMPTOMS

- Sudden onset pruritic, urticarial lesions, often on abdomen
- Progresses into generalized, bullous eruption sparing face, palms, and soles
- Spontaneous regression within weeks to months postpartum

ETIOLOGY

- Autoimmune disease. Autoantibodies bind to basement membrane zone
- Complement cascade activated
- Inherited predisposition, associated with HLA-DR3 and HLA-DR4 antigens

TREATMENT

- Topical corticosteroids, antipruritics, systemic steroids

FETAL EFFECTS

- Increased preterm birth
- Neonatal herpes gestationis reported in 10% of cases

RECURRENCE

- Recurrence may occur with menses, oral contraceptive use, and subsequent pregnancies.

IMPETIGO HERPETIFORMIS

SIGNS AND SYMPTOMS

- Erythematous patches with marginal pustules in groin, axilla, and neck
- Lesions expand with new pustules forming at leading edges
- Fever, nausea, vomiting, diarrhea commonly seen
- Elevated WBC and ESR
- Persists for weeks to months postpartum

ETIOLOGY

- Unknown

TREATMENT

- Antibiotics, oral corticosteroids

FETAL EFFECTS

- Maternal sepsis is common from secondary infection.
- Increased risk of fetal morbidity and mortality associated with placental insufficiency.

RECURRENCE

- May occur in subsequent pregnancies

CHAPTER 4

Gynecology

Jeannine Rahimian, MD, MBA
Malini Anand, MD
Caroline M. Colin, MD, MS
Chai Lin Hsu, MD
Milena M. Weinstein, MD
Judith A. Mikacich, MD

Definitions

- Normal menstrual cycle:
  - Interval 28 ± 7 days
  - Length 4 ± 2 days
  - Blood loss 60 ± 20 mL
- Metrorrhagia: Bleeding between cycles or prolonged duration of menses
- Menorrhagia: Heavy flow >80 mL
- Polymenorrhea: Cycle interval <21 days
- Oligomenorrhea: Cycle interval >35 days

DIFFERENTIAL DIAGNOSIS

- Anovulatory cycles:
  - Polycystic ovarian syndrome, endocrine disorders, hyperprolactinemia, estrogen-secreting tumors
- Uterine:
  - Endometrial polyp, hyperplasia, cancer, atrophy
  - Fibroids, endometriosis, adenomyosis, chronic endometritis
- Cervical:
  - Cancer, polyp, cervicitis, fibroid
- Pregnancy:
  - Threatened abortion, ectopic, gestational trophoblastic disease
- Vaginal:
  - Trauma, atrophy, foreign body, atrophic vaginitis
- Blood dyscrasias:
  - von Willebrand, leukemia, idiopathic thrombocytopenia purpura
- Systemic diseases:
  - Thyroid, adrenal, liver, renal
- Iatrogenic:
  - Anticoagulants, sex steroids, corticosteroids, intrauterine device (IUD)

DIAGNOSIS

HISTORY

Age, pattern of bleeding, precipitating factors, personal or family history of bleeding disorders, current medications

PHYSICAL

Vital signs, vagina, cervix, uterus, rectum, thyroid, evidence of hyperandrogenism (hirsutism, acne, acanthosis nigricans)

DIAGNOSTIC TESTS

- CBC, hCG, coagulation profile
- Pelvic ultrasound:
  - Fibroids, pelvic tumors, polyps
- Endometrial biopsy:
  - Hyperplasia, cancer
- Pap smear:
  - Cervical dysplasia, cancer

- Saline infusion sonohysterogram:
  - Endometrial polyp, submucosal fibroid
- Hysteroscopy:
  - Endometrial polyp, submucosal fibroid, hyperplasia, cancer
- Gonorrhea, chlamydia, wet mount, bacterial cultures:
  - Cervicitis, vaginitis

TREATMENT

ANOVULATORY CYCLES

- **Medical treatment**: Nonsteroidal anti-inflammatory drugs (NSAIDs), oral contraceptives, Depo-Provera, levonorgestrel IUD (Mirena)
- **Surgical management**: Endometrial ablation, hysterectomy
- **GnRH agonist**

FIBROIDS

- **Medical treatment**: NSAIDs, oral contraceptives, Depo-Provera, levonorgestrel IUD (Mirena)
- **Surgical management**: Hysteroscopy myomectomy, abdominal myomectomy, hysterectomy
- **GnRH agonist** (Depo-Lupron) can reduce fibroid size up to 40%
- **Uterine artery embolization:**
  - Reduces size of fibroids, blood loss, and pain.
  - Side effects are postoperative pain and fever, increased vaginal discharge.
  - Requires preprocedural MRI and MRA.
  - Fibroids >8 cm less effective.
  - Not indicated for women desiring future fertility.

ENDOMETRIAL POLYP

- Hysteroscopic resection
- Rarely malignant

ADENOMYOSIS

- **Medical treatment**: NSAIDs, oral contraceptives
- **Surgical management**: Hysterectomy
- **GnRH agonist** (Depo-Lupron)

▶ VAGINAL AND VULVAR INFECTIONS

Most common cause of vaginal and vulvar infections are bacterial vaginosis, candidiasis, and trichomonas vaginalis. See Table 4-1 for a comparison of these infections.

Bacterial Vaginosis

- Anaerobic bacteria (*Gardnerella vaginalis*) replace normal lactobacilli
- Symptoms: Thin, homogenous, gray-white discharge. Odor is fishy, often increased after intercourse

TABLE 4–1. **Characteristics of Vaginal Infections**

	DISCHARGE APPEARANCE	DISCHARGE pH	KOH "WHIFF TEST"	MICROSCOPY
Normal	White, clear	3.8–4.2	Negative	Normal epithelial cells
Bacterial vaginosis	Thin, gray-white	>4.5 (positive nitrazine test)	Positive	Clue cells, saline slide
Candidiasis	Thick, white, "cottage-cheese"	<4.5	Negative	Hyphae, budding yeast, KOH slide
Trichomonas	Green-yellow, frothy	>4.5 (positive nitrazine test)		Flagellated protozoan, saline slide

- Diagnosis: Vaginal pH 5–6, clue cells, positive "whiff" test with potassium hydroxide (KOH)
- Treatment: Oral or intravaginal metronidazole, oral or intravaginal clindamycin

Candidiasis

- Overgrowth of fungi (*Candida albicans or Candida glabrata*)
- Symptoms: Thick, white discharge, itching, burning, dysuria, dyspareunia
- Diagnosis: Vaginal pH 4–5, red vagina or vulva, hyphae and budding yeast on potassium hydroxide microscopy
- Treatment: Topical antifungal medication (e.g., miconazole, butoconazole), oral fluconazole

▶ SEXUALLY TRANSMITTED DISEASES

Trichomonas vaginalis

- Protozoan which lives in vagina, urethra, and Skene duct
- Sexually transmitted
- Symptoms: None in 50%. May have itching, burning, malodorous discharge, dysuria, dyspareunia
- Diagnosis: Vaginal pH >4.5, yellow green, thin discharge, red vulva, **strawberry patches on cervix** or vagina, flagellated protozoan on saline microscopy
- Treatment: Oral or intravaginal metronidazole. Sexual partners should be treated

Chlamydia

- Obligate intracellular parasite, *Chlamydia trachomatis*
- May cause cervicitis, urethritis, salpingitis, pelvic inflammatory disease, infertility, chronic infection, pelvic pain, **Fitz-Hugh Curtis syndrome**
- Symptoms: Often asymptomatic, mucopurulent discharge
- Diagnosis: Endocervical culture
- Treatment: Doxycycline or azithromycin; screening for other sexually transmitted diseases (STDs) mandatory when *Chlamydia* diagnosed

Gonorrhea

- Gram-negative intracellular diplococcus, *Neisseria gonorrhea*
- Infertility results in 15% after one episode and 75% after three episodes
- Symptoms: Purulent discharge, Bartholin gland abscess, urinary frequency, dysuria, asymptomatic
- Diagnosis: Endocervical culture, Gram stain
- Treatment: Ceftriaxone, cefixime, ofloxacin, levofloxacin, ciprofloxacin should also treat for *Chlamydia trachomatis*

Syphilis

- Anaerobic bacteria, spirochete *Treponema pallidum*
- Primary syphilis:
  - Painless, hard ulcer
  - Heals within 2–6 weeks
- Secondary syphilis:
  - Systemic disease, hematogenous spread
  - Diagnosed 6 weeks to 6 months after primary infection
  - Bilateral red macules and papules over palms and sides of feet
  - Vulvar condyloma lata
- Latent syphilis:
  - Optic atrophy, generalized paresis, aortic aneurysm, tabes dorsalis, gummas
  - Diagnosed 4–20 years after primary infection
- Diagnosis: Dark field examination, RPR, FTA
- Treatment: Penicillin G

Genital Herpes

- Herpes simplex virus type 1 (HSV 1) and type 2 (HSV 2).
- Symptoms: Unilateral recurrences in same location, average duration 7 days. Prodromal phase may include paresthesia, vulvar burning, tenderness, pruritus.
- Diagnosis: Vesicles visualized, viral culture from vesicle, **Tzanck smear** (scraping of ulcer shows giant cells).
- Treatment: Local anesthetic to reduce pain. Topical or oral antivirals reduce duration of shedding and time to healing.

Human Immunodeficiency Virus (HIV)

- Testing requires informed consent
- Symptoms (acute infection): Fever, adenopathy, pharyngitis, myalgias, rash
- Diagnosis: Enzyme immunoassay (ELISA) for screening, confirmed with Western blot or immunofluorescence assay
- Treatment: Goal is to suppress viral load, improve quality of life, restore immune function

Chancroid

- Nonmotile, anaerobic, gram-negative rod, *Haemophilus ducreyi*.
- Symptoms: Papule evolves into pustule, then **painful ulcer**, with gray, necrotic exudate. Tissue trauma must be present prior to infection (bacteria cannot penetrate skin). Tender inguinal adenopathy (bubo) in 50%.

- Diagnosis: Aspirated pus sent for culture, Gram stain.
- Treatment: Azithromycin, ceftriaxone, ciprofloxacin, erythromycin.

Lymphogranuloma Venereum

- Chronic infection of lymphatic tissue by *Chlamydia trachomatis*
- Occurs in tropical climate
- Symptoms: **Painless shallow ulcer**, adenopathy. Nodes can become enlarged and adherent to skin. **Groove sign**, depression between two lymph groups may be seen. Untreated, can progress to fibrosis, elephantiasis
- Diagnosis: Complement fixation for *Chlamydia*
- Treatment: Doxycycline or erythromycin, aspiration of fluctuant nodes

Granuloma Inguinale (Donovanosis)

- Nonmotile, gram-negative encapsulated rod, *Calymmatobacterium granulomatis*
- Occurs in tropical climate
- Symptoms: **Painless nodule**, ulcerated with beefy-red appearance
- Diagnosis: Biopsy or Wright smear of ulcer base (**Donovan bodies** seen)
- Treatment: Doxycycline or trimethoprim-sulfamethoxazole

Condyloma Acuminatum

- More than 100 types of human papillomavirus
- Immunosuppression, diabetes, pregnancy, local trauma predispose to infection
- Diagnosis: Visual appearance or biopsy
- Treatment: Trichloroacetic acid, imiquimod, podophyllin

Molluscum Contagiosum

- Caused by poxvirus, spread by local contact.
- Symptoms: Asymptomatic, umbilicated lesions 1–5 mm in diameter.
- Diagnosis: Visual appearance or biopsy.
- Treatment: Self-limited. Treated with imiquimod or sequence of evacuation of caseous material, excision of nodule with curet and treatment of base with Monsel solution or trichloroacetic acid.

▶ VULVAR DYSTROPHIES AND DERMATOSES

Lichen Sclerosus

- Most common in postmenopausal women
- Atrophic disease of vulva, thinning of epithelium
- Symptoms: Intense, chronic pruritus
- Diagnosis: Pale parchment-like areas, thickened areas, eventual loss of the normal external genitalia architecture. Biopsy usually confirmatory
- Treatment: High potency steroids (clobetasol)

Squamous Cell Hyperplasia (Lichen Simplex Chronicus)

- Epidermal hyperplasia due to chronic scratching and rubbing.
- Symptoms: Pruritus.
- Diagnosis: Thickened, white epithelium. Biopsy shows elongation and widening of epidermal rete pegs (acanthosis).
- Treatment: Removal of original causative agent, antipruritic agents, high-potency steroid (clobetasol).
- Prognosis is excellent.

Lichen Planus

- Symptoms: Burning, insertional dyspareunia
- Diagnosis: Bright red, patchy lesions. White cells on wet preparation, biopsy
- Treatment: Steroids

Eczema

- May be allergic or irritant
- Scratching and rubbing can lead to squamous hyperplasia
- Treatment: Withdrawal of the causative agent; skin should be kept clean and dry; cotton undergarments; topical steroids initially helpful

Psoriasis

- Familial pattern
- Diagnosis: Silvery scales seen
- Treatment: Steroids, UV light, coal tar preparations (refer to dermatology)

Hidradenitis Suppurativa

- Obstruction of apocrine glands in vulva and axilla
- Common in early reproductive years
- Leads to multiple draining sinuses, abscesses, scarring of the vulvar skin
- Treatment: Meticulous cleaning, avoiding tight clothing and sweating. Low-androgenic oral contraceptives, antibiotics during prolonged outbreaks. Surgical resection if severe
- Recurrence common

▶ BENIGN VULVAR MASSES AND LESIONS

Sebaceous or Epidermal Inclusion Cysts

- Caused by inflammatory blockage of the sebaceous gland ducts
- Small, smooth masses containing cheesy, sebaceous material

Bartholin Gland Cyst

- Cystic dilation of obstructed Bartholin duct.
- Fluid sterile in >90% of cases.
- If infectious, usually polymicrobial.
- Abscess can develop rapidly:
    - Involves acute pain, dyspareunia, edema, cellulitis of surrounding tissue.
    - Can be drained, Word catheter placed.

- If recurrent, marsupialization should be performed.
- Severe cases require surgical excision of gland.

Cyst of the Canal of Nuck

- Accumulation of peritoneal fluid in peritoneum where round ligament inserts into labium majora.

Fibromas

- Mass arising from connective tissue and smooth muscle of vulva and vagina
- Most common in labia majora
- Excise if symptomatic

Lipomas

- Similar in appearance to fibromas, but softer and usually larger
- Derived from fat cells in subcutaneous tissue of the vulva

Hidradenomas

- Arises from the sweat glands of the vulva
- Treated with excision

Hemangiomas

- Rare malformations of blood vessels
- Often discovered in childhood
- Usually single, 1–2 cm in diameter

Syringoma

- Rare, cystic, asymptomatic benign tumor.
- Adenoma of eccrine sweat glands.
- Identical tumors are found in the eyelids.

Vulvar Endometriosis

- Rare, seen in 1 in 500 with endometriosis.
- Blue, red, or purple subcutaneous lesions.
- Symptoms of cyclic discomfort and enlargement of the mass with periods.
- May cause pain, introital dyspareunia.

▶ PELVIC SUPPORT DEFECTS

Pelvic Support

Levator ani muscles (pelvic diaphragm) are the primary support of the pelvis:

- Innervated by S2, S3, S4
- Divided into two parts: Diaphragmatic (iliococcygeus and coccygeus muscles) and pubovisceral (puborectalis and pubococcygeus muscles)

- Thickening of pelvic sidewall at insertion of ileococcygeus muscle is **arcus tendineus**

Endopelvic fascia:

- Three-dimensional ligamentous mesentery of connective tissue that envelops pelvic organs and connects them to pelvic sidewalls
- Composed of pubocervical and rectovaginal fasciae

Uterosacral, round, infundibulopelvic, and cardinal ligaments also provide support to pelvic organs.

CAUSES OF DEFECTS

- Mechanical (childbirth, chronic constipation, heavy lifting, high-impact athletic activity)
- Genetic
- Hormonal
- Nutritional
- Environmental (cigarette smoking)
- Surrounding musculature, somatic, and visceral innervation (vascular or neurogenic disorders)

EVALUATION OF PELVIC SUPPORT DEFECTS

- Symptoms of pressure, sensation of "something falling out," vaginal fullness, back pain, groin pain
- Prolapse divided into anterior, apical, or posterior compartments:
    - Anterior compartment: Cystocele, urethrocele
    - Posterior compartment: Rectocele, enterocele
    - Apical compartment: Uterine descensus, vault prolapse (posthysterectomy)
- Description of defects is by grading system (grades 0–4) or with pelvic organ prolapse quantitative (POP-Q)

TREATMENT OF PELVIC SUPPORT DEFECTS

PELVIC MUSCLE EXERCISE

- No proven utility of Kegel exercise on POP-Q staging.
- Instruct patients with feedback by digital examination.
- Biofeedback improves outcome.

PESSARY

- Types include ring, cube, Gellhorn, doughnut, Gehrung, inflatoball, Schatz
- Follow-up 2 weeks after initial fitting, then every 3 months in first year
- Highest degree of pessary discontinuation is within first 12 months
- Potential problems:
    - Falls out with Valsalva (try larger size or alternative type)
    - Pelvic pain (try smaller size)
    - Vaginal bleeding from abrasions (try smaller size, vaginal estrogen)
    - Urinary incontinence unmasked by correction of prolapse
    - Vaginal discharge or odor (Trimo-san gel can decrease odor)

SURGICAL PROCEDURES

LE FORT COLPOCLEISIS

- Obliteration of vagina
- For advanced prolapse in elderly, not sexually active woman
- Performed under spinal anesthesia, with or without uterus in situ
- 95% success rates

ANTERIOR OR POSTERIOR COLPORRHAPHY

- Anterior or posterior defect
- Placation of pubocervical fascia anteriorly, levator muscles posteriorly in midline
- Defect directed repair: Repaired anatomically, precisely identifying fascial defects

PARAVAGINAL REPAIR

- Anterior or posterior defect
- Up to 85% of cystoceles originate from the lateral detachment
- Abdominal or laparoscopic reattachment of pubocervical fascia to arcus tendineus
- Complications: Rare urinary retention, hesitancy, abdominal straining

McCALL CULDOPLASTY

- For apical defect, usually performed with vaginal hysterectomy
- Plication of uterosacral ligaments, reefing posterior peritoneum of cul-de-sac
- Complications: Injury or kinking of ureter

UTEROSACRAL SUSPENSION

- Reattachment of uterosacral ligaments to vaginal apex with permanent sutures
- Vaginal or laparoscopic approach
- 87–90% success rates
- Complications: Ureteral injury rate 11% (requires cystoscopy)

ILEOCOCCYGEUS SUSPENSION

- Fixation of vaginal apex to fascia of ileococcygeus muscle, just anterior to ischial spine
- 95% success rate
- Complications: 14% rate of prolapse at other sites, loss of vaginal length

SACROSPINOUS FIXATION

- Fixation of vaginal apex to sacrospinous ligaments (unilateral or bilateral) with permanent sutures
- 70–99% success rate
- Complications: 20% anterior compartment prolapse, hemorrhage, vaginal shortening, sexual dysfunction, buttock pain, if unilateral fixation vaginal apex deviates to one side

SACRAL COLPOPEXY

- Placement of mesh (Mersilene, Prolene, Gortex) to bridge vaginal apex and sacral promontory
- Abdominal or laparoscopic approach

- >90% success rate
- Complications: 1–2% risk of catastrophic hemorrhage, mesh erosion

DIAGNOSIS AND EVALUATION

HISTORY

- Complete medical and surgical history is important
- Urology: Voiding diary with time and volume of spontaneous voids
- Medications that affect lower urinary tract:
    - Benzodiazepines: Secondary incontinence
    - Alcohol: Secondary incontinence and diuresis
    - Anticholinergic drugs: Impair detrusor contractility, lead to voiding difficulty, overflow incontinence
    - α-adrenergic agonist: Increase outlet resistance, lead to voiding difficulty
    - α-blockers: Decrease urethral closure, lead to stress incontinence
    - Calcium channel blockers: Voiding difficulty and incontinence
    - ACE-inhibitors: Chronic cough leads to increased stress incontinence

LABORATORY

- Complete urinalysis and urine culture

PHYSICAL EXAM

- Assess estrogen status.
- Neurological assessment: "Anal wink" and bulbocavernosus reflex, evidence of intact sacral reflex center.
- Q-tip test: Maximum straining angle >30° is urethral hypermobility.
- Postvoid residual (PVR): Normal is <50 mL, abnormal if >200 mL.
- Stress test: Patient coughs with full bladder in supine and standing positions.

URODYNAMIC TESTING

- **Filling cystometry**: Measurement of pressure to volume relationship of bladder during filling to detect detrusor overactivity. Simple cystometry done with manometer, complex cystometry done with electronic equipment.
- **Urethral closure pressure profile (UCP)**: Graph of urethral closure pressure along length of urethra (UCP = urethral pressure − intravesical pressure).
- **Abdominal leak-point pressure**: Intravesical pressure at which urine leakage occurs (increased abdominal pressure in absence of detrusor contraction).
- **Uroflowmetry**: Measurement of urine flow rate over time during voluntary voiding. Normal is void ≥200 mL at 10 mL/sec with PVR<50, otherwise obstructive voiding patterns are suspected.

Stress Urinary Incontinence (SUI)

- Involuntary leakage on effort, exertion, sneezing, coughing.
- Urodynamic stress incontinence (USI): Observation of involuntary urine leakage during increased abdominal pressure in absence of detrusor contraction.

- Nonsurgical treatment options include:
    - Behavioral therapy (weight loss, smoking cessation, control of straining)
    - Kegels exercise
    - Biofeedback with electrophysiological signals
    - Vaginal and urethral devices (pessary, urethral patch or plug)
- Surgical procedures done after childbearing completed. Options listed below.

RETROPUBIC SUSPENSION

- Burch procedure:
    - Abdominal or laparoscopic approach
    - 70–90% success rates
    - Complications: Delayed voiding, cystitis, detrusor instability
- The Marshall-Marchetti-Krantz (MMK):
    - Tissue from vagina and endopelvic fascia attached to periosteum of posterior pubic symphysis
    - 82–95% success rates
    - Complications: 2–10% rate of osteitis pubis

SUBURETHRAL SLING

- Synthetic slings (tension-free vaginal tape):
    - Polypropylene mesh
    - Success rate 81% at 7 years
    - Complications: Bladder perforation, voiding difficulties, detrusor instability, vessel injury, intestine injury
- Cadaveric or autologous sling:
    - Vaginal or abdominal approach.
    - Suburethral tissue secured to rectus fascia, iliopectineal line or bone anchors in pubic symphysis.
    - Success rates 80–95% (primary procedure), 70–85% (recurrent procedure).
    - Higher rate of complications: Incomplete bladder emptying, injury to lower urinary tract, recurrent urinary tract infections, vaginal or urethral erosion, urgency or urge incontinence.

PERIURETHRAL INJECTION

- For patients with good anatomical support, but malfunctioning urethra with low leak-point pressure
- Sterile bovine dermal collagen (Contigen), pyrolytical carbon-coated zirconium beads (Durasphere)
- Poorly conducted studies with variable outcomes

Overactive Bladder

- Urgency with or without incontinence, urinary frequency (>8 voids in 24 hours) and nocturia (>2 night voids)
- Detrusor overactivity is urodynamic observation of involuntary detrusor contractions during filling phase.
- Treatment options:
    - Behavioral therapy:
        - Lifestyle changes: Smoking cessation, weight reduction, management of fluid and food intake

- Bladder training: Scheduled voiding
- Kegel exercises: With or without biofeedback
- Electric stimulation: Of pelvic floor
  - Pharmacotherapy:
    - All drugs are anticholinergic, with side effects of dry mouth, constipation, increase in HR, drowsiness, blurry vision
    - Caution in patients with cardiac arrhythmias, narrow-angle glaucoma (precipitate rise in intraocular pressure)
    - Atrophic urethritis or vaginitis may be exacerbated
    - Success rates 60–80%

CHRONIC RETENTION OF URINE

- Replaces previous term of overflow incontinence
- Nonpainful bladder, remains palpable after patient has urinated
- May have incontinence
- Results from:
  - Obstruction at bladder outlet (pelvic organ prolapse, complication of incontinence surgery, urethral anomaly)
  - Physical or cognitive impairment (immobility, paralysis, muscular atrophy, dementia)

URETHRAL DIVERTICULA

- Symptoms: Stress incontinence, recurrent urinary tract infection, dysuria, dyspareunia, urgency
- Diagnosis: Palpable tender anterior vaginal wall mass, expression of pus from urethra
- Evaluation: Often multiple present, identified by voiding cystourethrography, cystourethroscopy, positive-pressure urethrography
- Treatment:
  - Transvaginal excision of diverticulum sac. Complications: Recurrent or persistent diverticula, urinary tract infection, fistula, stress incontinence
  - Marsupialization of diverticulum if very distal

▶ OVARIAN MASSES

History

- Age, general health, chronicity of growth
- Weight loss or gain, gastrointestinal symptoms, menstrual abnormalities

PHYSICAL EXAM

- Adnexal fullness, ascites, lymphadenopathy, signs of estrogen or masculinization

DIAGNOSTIC STUDIES

- Masses with the following ultrasound findings are suspicious:
  - Size ≥5 cm in postmenopausal or premenarchal patient
  - Size ≥10 cm

- Complex, solid, irregular, fixed, bilateral
- Size that has increased over time
- Associated with ascites
- Elevated CA-125:
  - Very elevated in postmenopausal cases should trigger investigation
  - In premenopausal cases, can be due to fibroids, pregnancy, pelvic inflammatory disease, hemorrhagic ovarian cyst, endometriosis, liver disease

DIFFERENTIAL DIAGNOSIS

NONOVARIAN ETIOLOGY

- Fibroid uterus
- Gastrointestinal causes (stool, gas, diverticulitis)
- Appendicitis
- Hernia
- Pregnancy (ectopic, intrauterine)
- Paratubal cyst
- Hydrosalpinx
- Tubo-ovarian abscess

OVARIAN MASSES

FUNCTIONAL OVARIAN CYST:

- Usually 2 mm to 15 cm
- Solitary or multiple
- Found in young, menstruating women
- Translucent, thin, walled with clear straw-colored fluid
- Asymptomatic or painful from distension of cyst wall or rupture
- Management: Observe for spontaneous resolution, repeat ultrasound every 4–8 weeks

CORPUS LUTEUM CYST:

- Usually 3–10 cm
- Cystic, occasionally hemorrhagic
- Can bleed 2–4 days after ovulation
- Asymptomatic or painful from intraperitoneal bleeding
- Management: Observe for spontaneous resolution or cystectomy

THECA LUTEIN CYST

- Often bilateral
- Due to prolonged stimulation of ovaries by endogenous or exogenous gonadotrophins or increased ovarian sensitivity to gonadotrophins
- Hyperreactio luteinalis: Multiple luteinized follicular cysts as seen occasionally with molar pregnancy or choriocarcinoma
- Management: Observation, usually regresses spontaneously

MATURE CYSTIC TERATOMA

- Composed of elements of three germ layers
- Most common neoplasm in teenagers and prepubertal girls

- Malignancy change very rare
- *Struma ovarii*: Overabundance of thyroid tissue (2–3% of teratomas)

ENDOMETRIOMA

- Found in 2/3 of women with endometriosis
- Ovaries commonly adherent to surrounding structures
- Management: Medical or surgical, depends on age, fertility, severity of symptoms

FIBROMAS

- Benign solid neoplasm of ovary
- Can be misdiagnosed as fibroids
- Arise from undifferentiated fibrous stroma of ovary
- Meig syndrome: Ovarian fibroma, ascites, hydrothorax. More likely if fibroma >6 cm
- Management: Surgical excision

▶ CHRONIC PELVIC PAIN

- Defined as persistent pelvic pain >6 months duration.
- Chronic pain may cause or exacerbate psychological disorders.
- Patients with chronic pain more often depressed, suffer from substance abuse, sexual dysfunction, and somatization disorders.

DIFFERENTIAL DIAGNOSIS

- Gastrointestinal: Inflammatory bowel disease, diverticulitis
- Urinary tract: Urinary infection, interstitial cystitis
- Psychosomatic illness
- Gynecologic:
  - Endometriosis, adenomyosis
  - Infectious: Chronic endometritis, salpingitis
  - Pelvic adhesions
  - Midcycle ovulation pain
  - Dysmenorrhea
  - Pelvic congestion syndrome

Diagnostic test options:

- Urinalysis and urine culture
- Cervical cultures for gonorrhea, *Chlamydia*, vaginal infections
- Gastrointestinal work up
- Psychiatric evaluation
- Trigger point injection with anesthetic agent
- Cystoscopy to rule out interstitial cystitis
- Laparoscopy to diagnose endometriosis

Medical management options:

- NSAIDs
- Continuous oral contraceptive pills
- GnRH agonists
- Medroxyprogesterone acetate injections (Depo-Provera)
- Narcotic analgesics and anxiolytics
- Antidepressants

Surgical management may include:

- Operative laparoscopy (adhesiolysis, destruction of endometriotic implants)
- Hysterectomy
- Presacral neurectomy

Presence of endometrial glands and stroma outside the uterus. Definitive diagnosis requires surgical identification of lesions.

Pathogenesis

Unknown pathogenesis, but theories include:

- Retrograde menstruation with transport of endometrial cells
- Metaplasia of coelomic epithelium
- Lymphatic or hematogenous dissemination

SYMPTOMS

- Pelvic pain, dysmenorrhea, dyspareunia, infertility, pain with defection
- Extent of disease has little correlation to severity of symptoms

PHYSICAL FINDINGS

There may be no signs on examination, but classic findings include:

- Tender nodules in posterior vaginal fornix
- Cervical motion tenderness
- Adnexal masses
- "Fixed" or frozen pelvis (due to adhesions)

DIAGNOSTIC TESTS

- Ultrasound: Endometrioma may be seen, or other causes to explain symptoms
- Laparoscopy: Direct visualization of lesions adequate for diagnosis, biopsy is not necessary. Lesions may be white, red, blue, brown, black

STAGING SYSTEM

- Classified as I (minimal), II (mild), III (moderate), IV (severe)
- Point system based on number, size, and location of implants and adhesions

TREATMENT

- Depends on severity of symptoms, age, desire for fertility.
- Medical management:
  - GnRH agonists with addback therapy
  - Medroxyprogesterone acetate
  - Continuous oral contraceptives
  - Danazol
  - Clomiphene citrate

- Surgical management
  - Eradication of implants by electrocautery, laser, excision
  - Hysterectomy
  - Oophorectomy

▶ BENIGN BREAST DISEASE

Fibrocystic Disease

- Definition: Fibrocystic breast changes with pain or nipple discharge. Not associated with increased risk of breast cancer.
- Symptoms: Luteal phase breast tenderness
- Diagnosis: Tender, lumpy breast tissue. Ultrasound can help confirm diagnosis.
- Treatment: NSAIDs. Controversial options are caffeine avoidance, vitamin E, evening primrose oil, danazol, tamoxifen, bromocriptine, oral contraceptives, GnRH agonists.

Fibroadenoma

- Definition: Benign solid tumor, containing glandular and fibrous tissue. Common in young women (age 20s). Transformation into cancer rare.
- Symptoms: Rare. Sensation of lump or mass
- Diagnosis: Firm, smooth, rubbery, discrete mass. Ultrasound can confirm diagnosis
- Treatment: Observation versus excision

Mastitis or Breast Abscess

- Definition: Infection of breast tissue, commonly with *Staphylococcus aureus* or *Streptococcus* species. Common in breast-feeding women.
- Symptoms: Breast pain, fever, myalgia
- Diagnosis: Tenderness, erythema, induration. Abscess palpated as discrete, fluctuant mass
- Treatment: Continued breast feeding or pumping; warm compresses; antibiotics; surgical drainage of abscess if not responsive to antibiotics.

Galactocele

- Definition: Cystic area containing milk. Commonly found after cessation of breast-feeding (up to 10 months).
- Symptoms: Mild pain
- Diagnosis: Mass discrete and very mobile. Needle aspiration confirms diagnosis
- Treatment: Needle aspiration, rarely excision

Fat Necrosis

- Definition: Often result of trauma to breast tissue. Consists of lipid-laden macrophages, scar tissue, and chronic inflammatory cells
- Symptoms: Pain
- Diagnosis: Tender, firm, ill-defined mass, may have surrounding ecchymosis. May show calcifications on mammography.
- Treatment: Expectant management versus excision

Tubular Adenoma

- Definition: Mass of ductal tissue, may increase in size during pregnancy and lactation
- Symptoms: Rare
- Diagnosis: Mobile, smooth mass. Biopsy required for diagnosis
- Treatment: Excision

Sclerosing Adenosis

- Definition: Hyperplastic changes of lobular tissue with increased fibrous tissue and interspersed glandular cells. No malignant potential.
- Symptoms: Rare
- Diagnosis: Identified on mammogram secondary to calcifications. Most common diagnosis of needle directed biopsy for abnormal mammogram findings
- Treatment: Excision

Diffuse Papillomatosis

- Definition: Formation of multiple papillomas in ducts
- Symptoms: Often present with bloody nipple discharge
- Diagnosis: Extremely small and difficult to palpate. Most (75%) located beneath nipple. May need galactography for diagnosis
- Treatment: Excisional biopsy of duct and surrounding tissue

▶ FIRST TRIMESTER PREGNANCY LOSS

Definitions

- Threatened abortion: Vaginal bleeding within first 20 weeks of gestation not ending in spontaneous abortion
- Inevitable abortion: Vaginal bleeding with cervical dilation, but no passage of tissue
- Incomplete abortion: Vaginal bleeding with cervical dilation and partial expulsion of products of conception
- Complete abortion: All fetal and placental tissue expelled, cervix closed, and vaginal bleeding decreasing
- Missed abortion: Fetal death with or without spotting, with no cervical dilation
- Septic abortion: Threatened, inevitable, or incomplete abortion with signs of uterine infection including elevated temperature, leukocytosis, lower abdominal tenderness, cervical motion tenderness, foul-smelling discharge

ETIOLOGY

- Chromosomal abnormality:
  - Accounts for 50% of first trimester miscarriages
  - Most common abnormality is autosomal trisomy
- Congenital anomaly:
  - Teratogen exposure
  - Diabetes

- Trauma
- Anatomical abnormalities
- Infection

RISK FACTORS

- Age
- Previous miscarriage
- Smoking (>10 cigarettes per day)
- Alcohol
- Drugs
  - NSAIDs
  - Cocaine
- Caffeine (>4–5 cups of coffee)

STATISTICS

- 30–40% risk of bleeding within first 20 weeks of gestation
- 50% of these cases end in spontaneous abortion
- Bleeding >3 days increases risk of abortions
- Cardiac activity at 6 weeks has 7% risk of abortion. At 8 weeks, risk is 2%

DIAGNOSIS

- Symptoms: Bleeding, cramping
- Quantitative hCG level
- Transvaginal probe ultrasound:
  - Gestational sac seen when hCG ≥1500 mIU/mL
  - Embryo with cardiac activity seen with hCG ≥13,000 mIU/mL
- Examination of cervical os
- Serum progesterone level <5 consistent with nonviable pregnancy
- Differential diagnosis:
  - Ectopic pregnancy
  - Incorrect dates
  - Threatened abortion
  - Physiological (implantation related)
  - Cervical or vaginal pathology

MANAGEMENT

- For all abortions:
  - RhoGAM administration if Rh negative (50 μg if <13 weeks, 300 μg >13 weeks)
  - Prophylactic antibiotics for surgical management (doxycycline 100 mg 1 hour prior and 200 mg post procedure)
- Threatened abortion:
  - No evidence of improved outcome with bed rest or restricted activities
- Inevitable or incomplete abortion:
  - Surgical dilation and curettage (see Abortion section)
  - Medical management misoprostol (see Abortion section)
  - Expectant management (70% complete without intervention)
- Complete abortion:
  - Ultrasonography to ensure that no retained products

The most common cause of spontaneous first trimester abortions is autosomal trisomy.

- Missed abortion:
  - Uterus should be evacuated within 5 weeks of suspected fetal death to prevent risk of consumptive coagulopathy
  - Surgical dilation and curettage (see Abortion section)
  - Medical management (see Abortion section)
- Septic abortion:
  - Laboratory assessment: CBC, urinalysis, chemistry and electrolyte panel, uterine discharge for culture and sensitivity
  - If septic, obtain blood cultures, chest x-ray, coagulation studies
  - IV antibiotics with broad coverage
  - Surgical uterine evacuation after antibiotics initiated

▶ ECTOPIC PREGNANCY

Majority of ectopic pregnancies occur in fallopian tube (95%), most commonly in the ampulla.

The ampulla of the fallopian tube is the most common site for ectopic pregnancies.

RISK FACTORS

- Majority do not have any risk factors
- Tubal pathology:
  - Pelvic inflammatory disease
  - Tubal surgery
- Previous ectopic pregnancy
- In utero diethylstilbestrol (DES) exposure (ninefold increased risk)
- Previous genital infections
- Infertility

DIAGNOSIS

- Symptoms:
  - Abdominal pain, amenorrhea, vaginal bleeding
  - >50% are asymptomatic prior to tubal rupture
- Physical examination:
  - Orthostatic hypotension
  - Adnexal or cervical tenderness
- Quantitative hCG: Rise <66% over 48 hours
- Pelvic ultrasound:
  - Absence of intrauterine gestational sac with hCG ≥2000 highly suggestive
  - Visualization of adnexal gestational sac or complex adnexal mass
- Curettage can be done for diagnostic purposes
- Differential diagnosis: Spontaneous abortion, ruptured corpus luteum cyst, threatened abortion, heterotopic pregnancy, appendicits, diverticulitis, adnexal pathology

TREATMENT

- Rh-negative patients should be given RhoGAM injection
- **Surgical management:**
  - Laparoscopy versus laparotomy depends on hemodynamic status
  - Salpingectomy versus salpingostomy dependent on size, location
  - Plateau or rise in hCG after surgery consistent with persistent ectopic pregnancy

- **Medical management** with methotrexate:
  - Side effect: Stomatitis, gastritis, alopecia, elevated liver enzymes
  - Failure rate, 6–14%, dependent on ectopic size, hCG level
  - Expect decline in hCG of ≥15% from day 4 to 7
  - Follow up with weekly hCG until negative
- Contraindications to medical management:
  - Hemodynamically unstable
  - Noncompliant or unable to follow up
- Relative contraindication to medical management:
  - High hCG
  - Large size
  - Cardiac activity

Counseling

- Recurrence rate:
  - 15% after one ectopic pregnancy
  - 30% after two ectopic pregnancies
- Factors more likely to result in recurrent ectopic pregnancy or infertility:
  - History of infertility
  - Maternal age
  - Prior tubal damage

▶ RECURRENT PREGNANCY LOSS

Definition and Facts

- Defined as ≥3 consecutive pregnancy losses before 20 weeks
- Incidence is 0.4–1%

Etiology

GENETIC ABNORMALITIES

Fetus with abnormal karyotype:

- Usually error during gametogenesis, fertilization, division of fertilized ovum.
- Diagnosis is with karyotype of products of conception.

Parent with abnormal karyotype:

- 2–4% of patients with recurrent loss have balanced chromosomal rearrangement.
- Diagnosis is with karyotypes of both parents.

HORMONAL AND METABOLIC DISORDERS

LUTEAL PHASE DEFECT

- Progesterone deficiency from dysfunction of corpus luteum or inadequate response of endometrium to progesterone.
- Deficiency results in inadequate endometrial development to support blastocyst.
- Diagnosis: Mid-luteal peak progesterone <10 ng/mL or luteal phase endometrial biopsy shows ≥3 days discrepancy between expected and actual dating pattern.
- Treatment: Progesterone supplementation.

HYPERSECRETION OF LH (POLYCYSTIC OVARY SYNDROME)

- High LH levels gives increased risk of miscarriage.
- Diagnosis: Elevated LH on day 8 of cycle.

ENDOCRINE DISORDERS

- Poorly controlled diabetes
- Autoimmune thyroid disease

UTERINE ANATOMICAL ABNORMALITIES

- Bicornuate, septate, or didelphic uterus:
  - Septate is most common abnormality.
  - DES exposure may be associated with uterine anomaly and recurrent loss.
  - Diagnosis: Hysterosalpingogram or pelvic ultrasound.
  - Treatment for bicornuate or septate: Transfundal metroplasty, transcervical hysteroscopic resection of septum.
- Cervical incompetence associated with second trimester loss:
  - Diagnosis: Asymptomatic dilation of cervix
  - Treatment: Cervical cerclage
- Other anatomical abnormalities:
  - Asherman syndrome
  - Submucosal fibroids

INFECTIOUS

- Numerous agents (*Toxoplasma*, HSV, *Ureaplasma urealyticum*, *Mycoplasma*, *Listeria*, *Chlamydia*) postulated to cause spontaneous abortion
- No evidence that any infectious agents cause first trimester loss
- Bacterial vaginosis treatment in women with history of preterm delivery shown to be beneficial
- Diagnosis: Genital cultures

Thrombophilias

ACQUIRED THROMBOPHILIA: ANTIPHOSPHOLIPID SYNDROME

- Presence of Anticardiolipin antibody (ACL) or lupus anticoagulant (LAC).
- Unclear mechanism. May involve inhibition of prostacyclin production from endothelial tissue, thereby increasing level of thromboxane.
- May exist without other autoimmune disorder (primary) or with underlying autoimmune disease such as SLE (secondary).
- Diagnosis: Presence of LAC, and/or ACL IgG (or both), and one clinical feature:
  - Three or more early losses with no more than one live birth
  - Unexplained second or third trimester fetal death
  - Unexplained venous or arterial thrombosis (including stroke)
  - Autoimmune thrombocytopenia
  - Must meet laboratory criteria on ≥2 occasions, 6 weeks apart
- Testing for anyone with:
  - Unexplained fetal death or stillbirth
  - Recurrent pregnancy loss
  - Severe preeclampsia <34 weeks of gestation
  - Severe intrauterine growth restriction in second or early third trimester
- Treatment with aspirin, heparin.

INHERITED THROMBOPHILIAS

- Factor V Leiden, hyperhomocysteinemia, prothrombin G20210A mutation
- Diagnosis: Laboratory analysis for gene mutations
- Treatment: Unclear benefit

ENVIRONMENTAL FACTORS

- Smoking, alcohol, irradiation

IDIOPATHIC

- In 35–44%, no etiologic factor will be found

Evaluation of Recurrent Loss

- Start workup after two or three first trimester losses
- Evaluation warranted after any second trimester loss
- History: regarding cervical incompetence, exposure to toxins, thyroid disease, family history
- Physical exam including detection of hirsutism, galactorrhea, genital tract abnormalities
- Laboratory studies:
  - CBC, TSH, antithyroid antibodies
  - Day 8 LH, mid-luteal serum progesterone
  - Homocystine, anticardiolipin, lupus anticoagulant, activated protein C resistance.
- Other studies: Hysterosonogram, hysteroscopy, karyotype of parents

MNEMONIC FOR RECURRENT PREGNANCY LOSS

RIBCAGE
Radiation
Immune reaction or idiopathic
Bugs (infection)
Cervical incompetence
Anatomical anomaly (uterine septum)
Genetic (aneuploidy, balanced translocation)
Endocrine

▶ PERIOPERATIVE CARE

Informed Consent

Discussion and documentation of the following:

- Indication for procedure
- Explanation of procedure details
- Risks and benefits expected
- Unexpected findings or possible modifications

Preoperative Assessment

- Thorough medical and surgical history
- Complete physical exam

- Laboratory tests (CBC, blood type)
- Ensure that pap smear and mammogram screening are up-to-date
- Medical clearance in elderly or patient with history of medical problems

Special considerations in **elderly** population:

- May be taking multiple medications
- Greater coronary risk, cardiovascular morbidity, and mortality
- Risk of dehydration associated with bowel preparations
- Inadequate pain control increases risk of postoperative delirium

Postoperative Complications

FEVER

- Immediate (within hours): Drug fever (eosinophilia present), malignant hyperthermia, transfusion reaction
- Acute (within 1 week): Atelectasis, pneumonia, urinary tract infection, wound infection, deep vein thrombosis, thrombophlebitis, pulmonary embolism, myocardial infarction
- Subacute (1–4 weeks): Central venous catheter site, antibiotic associated diarrhea, medication reaction, deep vein thrombosis, pulmonary embolism
- Delayed (after 4 weeks): Viral infections, infection of implanted device

ILEUS

- Characterized by abdominal distention, absence of bowel sounds, generalized abdominal tympany.
- Usually within 48–72 hours.
- Abdominal x-ray shows generalized dilation and distention. May be similar findings in partial obstruction.
- Treatment: Expectant management, nasogastric tube if severe vomiting or distention, monitor electrolytes.

OBSTRUCTION

- Characterized by severe vomiting, abdominal pain, tympanic abdomen
- Often consequence of peritonitis or irritation resulting in adhesions
- Usually seen postoperative day 5 or 6
- Abdominal x-ray shows dilation and distention of small bowel with **air fluid levels** if completely obstructed
- Treatment: Conservative with nasogastric tube or surgical management

RESPIRATORY COMPLICATIONS

- Major complication, causing 30% of postoperative deaths within 6 weeks.
- **Atelectasis:** Airway collapse caused by splinting. Risk factors include chronic bronchitis, asthma, smoking, respiratory infections. Prevention is with smoking cessation, minimizing pain, incentive spirometer.
- **Pneumonia:** May follow atelectasis or vomiting. Treatment with antibiotics, deep breathing, coughing.

THROMBOEMBOLISM

- Most common in calf, can also occur in thigh or pelvis.
- Symptoms: Leg pain, asymmetry of calves, **Homans sign** (specific, not sensitive).

- Risk factors: Obesity, cancer, oral contraceptive use, diabetes, hypercoagulable state (protein C and S deficiencies, factor V Leiden mutation).
- Diagnosis: Contrast venography is gold standard.
- Treatment: Heparin, oral anticoagulant, subcutaneous low molecular weight heparin.
- Prevention: Subcutaneous heparin, pneumatic compression devices.

A positive Homans sign is a specific but not sensitive test for deep vein thrombosis.

POSTOPERATIVE INFECTION

- **Risk factors**: No antibiotic prophylaxis, field contamination, immune compromised, obesity, poor nutrition, low socioeconomic status, diabetes, prolonged operating time, anemia.
- **Wound infection**: Cellulitus, seroma, deep wound infections (surgical emergency if fascia not intact), necrotizing fascitis.
- **Urinary tract infection**: Foley catheters increase risk.
- **Cuff cellulitis**: Late fever, pelvic pain, discharge, mild leukocytosis.
- **Septic pelvic thrombophlebitis**: Presents 2–4 days after surgery with fevers, tachycardia, gastrointestinal upset, abdominal pain, palpable abdominal cord. Treatment with 7–10 days of heparin, broad spectrum antibiotics until afebrile for 48 hours.
- **Osteomyelitis pubis**: After retropubic urethral suspension, radical vulvectomy, pelvic exenteration. Presents 6–8 weeks after surgery with low-grade fevers, pain with ambulation, elevated ESR, positive blood or bone cultures.

▶ CRITICAL CARE

Toxic Shock Syndrome

- Caused by bacterial exotoxin, TSS toxin, produced by *Staphylococcus aureus*
- 50% of cases related to menses, tampon, diaphragm use
- Symptoms:
  - High fever (>38.9)
  - Diffuse macular rash
  - Desquamation 1–2 weeks after onset
  - Hypotension (SBP <90 mmHg)
  - Multiorgan involvement (≥3 systems: gastrointestinal, muscular, mucus membrane, renal, hepatic, hematologic, pulmonary, central nervous system)
- Laboratory findings: Elevated WBC, elevated bilirubin, elevated creatinine, prolonged PT, negative cerebrospinal fluid culture
- Treatment: Penicillin, supportive therapy
- Recurrence 30%. Prevention by minimizing tampon use
- Mortality rate 2–8% (due to respiratory distress, disseminated intravascular coagulation, intractable hypotension)

Septic Shock

- Caused by gram-positive and negative organisms
- Endotoxin leads to consumptive coagulopathy, complement activation
- Characterized by low systemic vascular resistance, high cardiac output
- Symptoms: Altered mental status, tachypnea, vomiting, diarrhea
- Diagnosis: Hypotension, oliguria, hypothermia, respiratory alkalosis
- Studies and tests: Blood cultures, complete blood count, liver and kidney function tests, coagulation profile, chest x-ray, arterial blood gas

■ Treatment: Stabilization, broad spectrum antibiotics, volume repletion, inotropic agent if needed

Hypovolemic Shock

■ Hypotension, tachycardia, weak pulse, pallor, diminished urinary output, peripheral vasoconstriction
■ Results from hemorrhagic cause (acute blood loss, ectopic pregnancy) or nonhemorrhagic causes (intestinal obstruction, vomiting, diarrhea)

Cardiogenic Shock

■ Findings similar to hypovolemic shock
■ Results from cardiac tamponade, pneumothorax, myocardial infarction, congestive heart failure

Acute Respiratory Distress Syndrome

■ Acute onset, severe lung disease
■ Injury to pulmonary epithelium and endothelium, increased vascular permeability
■ 80% associated with infection, trauma, aspiration
■ Severe hypoxemia unresponsive to oxygen therapy, pulmonary infiltrates
■ Treatment: Supportive therapy
■ Survival 60%

Central Monitoring

Peripheral artery cannulation:

■ Assessment of systemic arterial pressure in situation of hemodynamic instability
■ Placed in radial artery
■ Complications: Septicemia, local infection, embolization

Central venous pressure monitoring:

■ Assessment of fluid status
■ Placed from right internal jugular to right atrium
■ Complications: Pneumothorax

Swan-Ganz catheter

■ Helps prevent fluid overload, congestive failure, pulmonary edema
■ Measurement of pulmonary capillary wedge pressure
■ Complications: Sepsis, pulmonary infarction, balloon rupture
■ Infrequently used due to high complication rate and other available options

Pulmonary Embolism

■ Symptoms: Pleuritic chest pain, hemoptysis, dyspnea, tachycardia, tachypnea
■ Symptoms may be subtle or nonexistent
■ Diagnostic tests: ECG, arterial blood gas, spiral CT, ventilation perfusion lung scan. Gold standard is pulmonary angiography
■ Treatment: Anticoagulation, respiratory support, vena cava filter for prevention of recurrent emboli

Functional Assessment

- Cognitive function and depression should be assessed via:
  - Folstein Mini-Mental Status Examination
  - Short Portable Mental Status Questionnaire
  - Beck Depression Screen
- Physical exam should include vision and hearing assessment
- Issues to assess may include nutritional status, home safety, gait, and balance

Preventive Health Services

See Screening section (Chapter 7, Primary and Preventive Care) for review of recommended screening tests, intervals, immunizations.

Surgical Care of Geriatric Patient

Geriatric patients are at increased risk for surgical complications, such as:

- Nerve entrapment
- Hypothermia
- Fluid and electrolyte imbalance
- Thromboembolism

The following is important in the postoperative period:

- Analgesia dose adjustments to compensate for changes in drug metabolism and excretion. Medications commonly causing adverse reactions are:
  - Psychotropic medications
  - Diuretics
  - Cardiovascular agents
- Early ambulation and prophylaxis for thromboembolism
- Fall prevention

Contraindications

- Absolute: Bowel obstruction, ileus, peritonitis, intraperitoneal hemorrhage, diaphragmatic hernia, severe cardiorespiratory disease
- Relative: Extremes of body weight, inflammatory bowel disease, large abdominal mass, advanced intrauterine pregnancy

Complications

- Mortality rate 3–8 per 100,000
- Pneumoperitoneum:
  - Extraperitoneal insufflation with the Veress needle.
  - When recognized, should allow gas to escape and reinsert needle.
  - Usually resolves spontaneously.
  - Mediastinal emphysema causes ventilation difficulty.
  - Penetrating vessel injury may cause gas embolism and death recognized by "mill wheel" murmur over the precordium.

GYNECOLOGY

- Vessel injury:
    - Most common is inferior epigastric injury with trocar placement
    - Aorta or vena cava injury extremely rare
    - Increased risk in thin patients
- Bowel injury:
    - Direct trauma (trocar or Veress) or electrosurgical injury.
    - Burn injuries require resection of tissue around injury site.
    - Unrecognized injury presents with pain, fever, ileus.
- Bladder injury
    - Decrease risk with bladder drainage at start of case.
    - Trocar injury requires surgical repair.
    - Unrecognized injury presents with urinary ascites, abdominal pain, distention, fever, elevated creatinine.
- Ureteral injury:
    - Usually occur near cervix and uterosacral ligament.
    - Injury can be assessed with indigo carmine dye or cystoscopy.
    - Unrecognized injury presents with flank, pelvic, back or abdominal pain, fever, elevated creatinine.
- Nerve injury:
    - Result of inappropriate positioning or direct injury

▶ HYSTEROSCOPY

Contraindications

- Infection: Cervical, endometritis, pelvic inflammatory disease, salpingitis
- Cancer: Cervical, endometrial

Distending media

CARBON DIOXIDE

- Advantages: Can be done in office
- Disadvantages: Mixes with blood and obscures image, risk of emboli with flow rate greater than 100 mL/min

LACTATED RINGERS (LR) AND NORMAL SALINE (NS)

- Advantages: Safest of distending media
- Disadvantages: Cannot be used with monopolar electrosurgery, risk of fluid overload leading to pulmonary edema

GLYCINE AND SORBITOL

- Advantages: Can be used with monopolar electrosurgical devices.
- Disadvantages: Hypoosmolar, leads to increased vascular absorption, severe hyponatremia, increased risk of cerebral edema (female brain cells deficient in cation pumping mechanism)

HYSKON (DEXTRAN)

- Advantages: Doesn't mix with blood so provides excellent visualization
- Disadvantages: Risk of pulmonary edema, rare anaphylactic reaction

Complications

- Uterine perforation: Should evaluate with laparoscopy to identify extent of perforation, evaluate for bowel, bladder, vessel injury
- Bleeding: Especially if myometrial wall entered. Can tamponade with Foley catheter
- Complications due to distending media (fluid overload, pulmonary edema, cerebral edema, embolism)

▶ CONTRACEPTION

Definitions

- Birth Rate: Number of live births per 1000 population
- Fertility rate: Number of live births per 1000 women aged 15–44 (more sensitive measure of reproductive activity)
- Theoretical effectiveness: Pregnancy rate among those who use method correctly each time of use
- Actual effectiveness: Pregnancy rate with typical use of method

METHODS OF CONTRACEPTION

See Table 4-2 for failure rates for each contraception method. Factors to discuss with patients regarding contraceptive options:

- Efficacy
- Future fertility and reversibility
- Convenience
- Changes in bleeding pattern
- Protection against sexually transmitted diseases
- Risks and complications
- Cost

COITUS INTERRUPTUS

- Withdrawal of penis before ejaculation
- Advantages: Nonhormonal, no cost, easy
- Disadvantages: High failure rate

NATURAL FAMILY PLANNING

- Periodic abstinence or "rhythm" method
- Can be via calendar method, temperature, cervical mucus assessment, symptothermal, or combination

LACTATIONAL AMENORRHEA (LAM)

- Fertility is low within 6 months postpartum if breast-feeding exclusively
- Pregnancy rate is 1% at 6 months, 7% at 12 months

MALE CONDOM

- Advantages: Protection against sexually transmitted infections, nonhormonal
- Disadvantages: High failure rate

TABLE 4-2. **Failure Rates of Contraceptive Methods**

Contraceptive Method	Perfect Use (%)	Typical Use (%)
Abstinence	0	0
No method	85	85
Spermicide	6	26
Natural family planning		25
Symptothermal	2	
Cervical mucus	3	
Calendar	9	
Withdrawal	4	19
Male condom	3	14
Diaphragm	6	18
Mini-pill	0.5	3–6
Combination pill	0.1	3
Depo-Provera	0.3	0.3
Copper IUD	0.6	0.8
Levonorgestrel IUD	0.1	0.1
Sterilization (male)	0.1	0.15
Sterilization (female)	0.5	0.5

DIAPHRAGM

- Advantages: Nonhormonal
- Disadvantages: Inconvenient, increased risk of urinary tract infection, toxic shock syndrome
- Contraindications: Not for use for those at risk for or with HIV

PROGESTIN ONLY PILL

- Advantages: Can be used if unable to take estrogen
- Disadvantages: Increased break through bleeding, high failure rates

ORAL CONTRACEPTIVES

- Advantages: Reduction in dysmenorrhea, menorrhagia, ovarian cancer, endometrial cancer, pelvic inflammatory disease

- Disadvantages: Requires daily use, may increase blood pressure
- Absolute contraindications:
  - History of thromboembolic event or stroke
  - Liver disease
  - Estrogen-dependent tumor
  - Women ≥35 who smoke
  - Undiagnosed abnormal bleeding
- Relative contraindications
  - Poorly controlled hypertension
  - Seizure medication use
  - History of migraine headache

CONTRACEPTIVE PATCH

- Combination hormone contraceptive
- Advantages: Convenient weekly use, effective
- Disadvantages: Visible patch, breast tenderness, nausea, headache

CONTRACEPTIVE VAGINAL RING

- Advantages: Lower hormone dose, convenience, rapid return to ovulation
- Disadvantages: Vaginal discharge

INJECTABLE DEPOT MEDROXYPROGESTERONE ACETATE (DMPA)

- Advantages: High efficacy, reduction of endometrial cancer and pelvic inflammatory disease
- Disadvantages: Fertility may be delayed up to 18 months after discontinuation, irregular bleeding, effects on bone density, acne, headache, depression

COPPER INTRAUTERINE DEVICE (CIUD)

- Advantages: Long-term, convenient, high efficacy, easily reversible
- Contraindication: Current vaginal infection, at high risk for sexually transmitted infection

LEVONORGESTREL IUD

- Advantages: High efficacy, long-term, convenient, easily reversible, decreased menstrual flow, improvement of dysmenorrhea
- Disadvantages: Irregular spotting
- Contraindication: Current vaginal infection, at high risk for sexually transmitted infection

STERILIZATION

- Most common method of contraception (male and female combined)
- Advantages: Effective, easy to use, reduction of ovarian cancer risk
- Disadvantages: Ectopic pregnancy, regret, potential surgical complications

POSTCOITAL CONTRACEPTION

- Should be taken within 72 hours of intercourse
- Plan B (levonorgestrel):

Sterilization is the most common method of contraception in the United States.

- - Mechanism uncertain. Interrupts before implantation
    - 1% failure (pregnancy rate)
  - Yuzpe method:
    - Ethinyl estradiol 100 μg and levonorgestrel 0.5 mg
    - Nausea and vomiting is common side effect
    - 3% failure (pregnancy rate)
  - Mifepristone (RU-486)
    - Prevents implantation
    - 1% failure (pregnancy rate)

▶ INDUCED ABORTION

Rh D–negative patients should receive RhoGAM injection, regardless of abortion route.

Menstrual Extraction (<7 weeks)

- Early manual curettage with 6 mm cannula and syringe
- Follow-up with hCG to ensure completion and not ectopic pregnancy

Suction Curettage (<13 weeks)

- Preoperative gonorrhea and chlamydia recommended.
- Misoprostol or laminaria placement several hours prior decreases uterine perforation risk.
- Saline floating test ensures villi presence.
- Prophylactic antibiotics decreases infection risk.
- Complications: Pain, bleeding, infection, retained products.

Dilation and Evacuation (>13 weeks)

- Laminaria placement for several hours or overnight.
- Performed with long forceps, large bore vacuum cannula.
- Intraoperative ultrasound recommended if >14 weeks.
- Prophylactic antibiotics decreases infection risk.
- Complications: Coagulopathy, bleeding, uterine perforation.

Medical Abortion

Complication of all methods is incomplete abortion, heavy bleeding.

METHOTREXATE PLUS PROSTAGLANDIN

- If pregnancy ≤56 days
- Methotrexate intramuscular, misoprostol day 5–7
- 92% completion
- Takes longer but less expensive than mifepristone

MIFEPRISTONE (RU-486) PLUS PROSTAGLANDIN

- If pregnancy ≤49 days
- Mifepristone 600 mg, day 1; misoprostol day 2–3

- 92–98% completion
- Contraindications: Severe asthma, chronic renal failure, unable to follow up, long-term steroid use

INTRAVAGINAL PROSTAGLANDIN

- Misoprostol placed in vagina
- 82–95% completion
- Contraindications: severe asthma, unable to follow up

Stages of Response

EXCITEMENT

- Associated with deep breathing, increase in heart rate, increase in blood pressure
- Engorgement of breasts, labia majora and minora, clitoris
- **Sex flush**: Maculopapular rash on breasts and chest
- Vaginal transudative lubricant

PLATEAU

- Culmination of excitement phase
- Vasocongestion throughout body
- **Orgasmic platform**: Vasocongestion in lower third of vagina
- Vagina lengthens, upper vagina dilates

ORGASM

- Release of sexual tension
- Myotonic response involving muscles of entire body (especially vagina, uterus, anal sphincter)
- Sexual gratification associated with nerve endings in clitoris, mons pubis, labia

RESOLUTION

- Return of physiologic state to preexcitement level
- Total resolution time up to 30 minutes
- Usually associated with feeling of personal satisfaction and well-being
- Refractory period more common and more lengthy in males than females

Sexual Function Disorders

LOSS OF DESIRE AND AROUSAL (HYPOACTIVE SEXUAL DESIRE DISORDER)

- Most common sexual dysfunction
- May result from age, dyspareunia, medications, life stressors
- Treatment: Counseling, discontinuation of medication, lifestyle changes (exercise, smoking cessation, decrease alcohol intake), hormone therapy

ANORGASMIA

- 10–15% have never experienced an orgasm
- 25–35% have difficulty reaching orgasm
- Discern if able to have orgasm with masturbation, oral intercourse, vaginal intercourse, or not at all
- May result from medications (e.g., SSRIs)
- Treatment: Counseling, masturbatory techniques

VAGINISMUS

- Involuntary spasm of vaginal introitus and levator ani muscles
- Penile penetration painful or impossible
- May have difficulty inserting tampon or with vaginal examination
- Due to sexual abuse, painful episiotomy repairs, severe vaginitis, aversion to sexuality
- Treatment: Self-dilation, counseling, psychotherapy

DYSPAREUNIA

- Pain with intercourse
- Delineate if during insertion, mid-vagina with thrusting or deep penetration
- Causes: Poor lubrication, urethritis, cystitis, previous laceration or episiotomy, pelvic inflammatory disease, episiotomy, hymen, Bartholin gland abscess, atrophic
- Treatment: Treating infection, attempting alternate positions, lubrication, opening of hymen, incision or excision of Bartholin gland abscess

CHAPTER 5

Reproductive Endocrinology and Infertility

Susan Sarajari, MD, PhD
Jeannine Rahimian, MD, MBA
Gayane Ambartsumyan, MD
Mor Tzadik, MD, MS
Judith A. Mikacich, MD
Caroline M. Colin, MD

► SEXUAL DIFFERENTIATION

- Urogenital tract develops from differentiation of wolffian and müllerian ducts.
- SRY gene on Y chromosome causes gonad to develop into testes.
- Antimüllerian hormone or müllerian inhibiting factor:
  - Produced by Sertoli cells of testis
  - Causes regression of ipsilateral müllerian ducts
- Testosterone:
  - Secreted by fetal testes
  - Stimulates wolffian duct differentiation
- Dihydrotestosterone (DHT):
  - Product of 5α-reductase conversion of testosterone
  - Responsible for development of male external genitalia

Females

- Müllerian ducts give rise to:
  - Fallopian tubes
  - Uterus
  - Upper vagina
- Wolffian ducts remain in vestigial form.
- External genitalia:
  - Genital tubercle becomes the clitoris.
  - Genital swellings become the labia majora.
  - Genital folds become the labia minora.

Males

- Wolffian duct gives rise to:
  - Epididymides
  - Vasa deferentia
  - Seminal vesicles
  - Ejaculatory ducts
- Müllerian ducts regress.
- External genitalia:
  - Genital tubercle becomes the glans penis.
  - Genital swellings fuse to become the scrotum.
  - Genital folds become the shaft of the penis.

► MÜLLERIAN TRACT DEVELOPMENT

- Müllerian ducts elongate caudally and meet in midline.
- At 12 weeks, caudal portion of müllerian ducts fuse to form uterovaginal canal.
- Internal canalization and resolution of septum between ducts occurs by 20 weeks.
- Cranial portion of müllerian ducts develop into fimbria and fallopian tubes.
- Development of gonads is separate from müllerian system.

Abnormal Müllerian Development

- Müllerian tract is close to mesonephric development, so renal anomalies seen in 20–30% of those with müllerian defects.

VAGINAL DEFECTS

- Transverse vaginal septum:
  - Failure of fusion or canalization of müllerian ducts or urogenital sinus
  - Can occur at various levels in vagina, upper, middle, or lower
- Longitudinal vaginal septum:
  - Commonly occur with didelphic uterus
  - May be partial or complete
  - Often associated with renal defects
- Vaginal agenesis (Mayer-Rokitansky-Küster-Hauser syndrome):
  - See Amenorrhea section for details.

UTERINE ABNORMALITIES

- Uterine anomalies occur in 2–4% with normal reproduction
- Septate uterus:
  - Most common uterine abnormality (90%).
  - Defect of canalization or resorption of septum between müllerian ducts.
  - External surface of uterus appears normal.
  - Miscarriage rate may be higher with long septum.
- Bicornuate:
  - Accounts for 5% of cases.
  - Due to partial fusion of ducts.
  - Fundus indented ≥1 cm. Usually with normal vagina.
  - Separation of horns can be minimal, partial, complete.
  - Pregnancy outcome similar to general population, but increased abnormal presentation rate.
- Didelphic uterus:
  - Accounts for 5% of cases.
  - Müllerian ducts fail to fuse.
  - Presence of two cervices (bicollis) is common.
  - Less frequently seen is duplication of vagina, bladder, urethra, anus.
- Unicornuate uterus:
  - One side normal fallopian tube and cervix, other side abnormal
  - Higher incidence of endometriosis, infertility, preterm labor, abnormal presentation
  - 40% associated with renal abnormalities

▶ PEDIATRIC AND ADOLESCENT GYNECOLOGY

Puberty

- Hypothalamic pituitary ovarian (HPO) axis:
  - Quiescent until puberty
  - Activation results in GnRH secretion from hypothalamus and FSH, LH from pituitary gland.
- Hypothalamic pituitary adrenal (HPA) axis:
  - Produces adrenal androgens
  - Responsible for development of pubic hair (adrenarche)

Classic sequence of puberty:

- Thelarche: Breast and areolar development
- Adrenarche: Pubic hair development
- Peak growth spurt: Growth hormone secretion continues
- Menarche: Usually 2–3 years after thelarche

Tanner staging system of breast and pubic hair development:

- Stage I: Prepubertal breast and pubic hair
- Stage II: Breast bud, sparse hair along labia
- Stage III: Elevation of breast, hair becomes darker, coarser, curlier
- Stage IV: Areola develops mound above breast, mid-escutcheon hair
- Stage V: Breast develops adult contour, female escutcheon

Birth to Menarche

HISTORY AND PHYSICAL

- History should be obtained from child rather than parent if possible.
- Vulva and vagina examination in "frog-leg" or "knee-chest" positions.
- Rectal examination to confirm presence of uterus.
- Cultures can be obtained via saline moistened swabs inserted through hymenal ring or insertion of saline through hymenal ring then asking child to cough.

VULVOVAGINITIS

- Most common problem in prepubertal girls
- Risk factors:
    - Close proximity of vagina to rectum
    - Suboptimal hygiene
    - Neutral pH
    - Atrophic vaginal mucosa
- Differential diagnosis:
    - Nonspecific (75% of cases): Cultures reveal normal flora.
    - Candida:
        - Most often when in diapers or after antibiotics
        - Can accompany lichen sclerosus
        - Treat with antifungal cream
    - Shigella:
        - Very uncommon
        - Associated with recent history of diarrhea, persistent bloody, purulent vaginal discharge
        - Treat with trimethoprim sulfamethoxazole
    - Pinworm:
        - Accompanied by perianal pruritus
        - Treat with mebendazole
    - Sexually transmitted infections.
    - Contact dermatitis caused by irritant exposure (soaps, detergents).
    - Foreign body with toilet tissue most common.

Most cases of vulvovaginitis in young girls is nonspecific with culture reveal normal flora.

LICHEN SCLEROSUS

- Inflammatory disease characterized by itching and soreness of vulva, perianal, perineal skin.
- Sclerotic, atrophic plaque with hourglass or keyhole appearance.
- Subepithelial hemorrhage may be present and does not connote sexual abuse.
- Secondary infection common.
- Biopsy not usually necessary.
- Treat with clobetasol propionate twice daily then tapered.

LABIAL AGGLUTINATION

- Fusion of labia minora edges.
- Results from local irritation and scratching.
- Treat with estrogen cream and weak steroid cream.

TRAUMA AND SEXUAL ABUSE

- Traumatic injuries most commonly anterior, extending to mons pubis
- Sexual abuse often involves posterior vagina or anus. Laceration of posterior hymen between 3 and 9 o' clock suspicious
- Straddle injury:
  - Usually due to fall onto bicycle bar, getting in or out of pool or bathtub.
  - Evaluate under anesthesia if necessary.
  - Anorectal injuries rare but must be ruled out.
- Vulvar hematoma managed conservatively. Surgical drainage if expanding or impeding urination

OVARIAN MASSES

- Ovarian torsion should be suspected if pain and nausea present. Laparoscopy when suspected.
- Germ cell tumors are 60% of ovarian masses in children. See Chapter 6, Oncology.

Adolescent Issues

MENSTRUAL CYCLE ABNORMALITIES

- Amenorrhea—see Amenorrhea section.
- Oligomenorrhea:
  - First 12–18 months after menarche usually anovulatory cycles
  - Sports, eating disorders, thyroid disorders
  - Polycystic ovarian syndrome—see polycystic ovarian syndrome section.
- Menorrhagia may be due to:
  - Anovulatory cycles
  - Blood dyscrasias: Thrombocytopenia purpura, von Willebrand disease
- "Female athlete triad" is amenorrhea, osteoporosis, disordered eating.

DYSMENORRHEA AND PELVIC PAIN

- Primary dysmenorrhea:
  - Painful menses without pelvic pathology.
  - Begins shortly after menarche.
  - Treatment is NSAIDS, hormonal contraceptives (oral, patch, vaginal ring).
- Secondary dysmenorrhea:
  - Painful menses with underlying pelvic pathology, such as fibroids, endometriosis, salpingitis.
  - Treatment is of underlying pathology.
- If pain noncyclic, look for other pelvic pathology via ultrasound.
- Dysmenorrhea is associated with premenstrual syndrome and symptoms of stress, anxiety, mood swings. Calcium supplementation may be helpful.

SEXUALITY AND CONTRACEPTIVE NEEDS

- Discuss abstinence as best protection against pregnancy and infection
- Annual sexually transmitted disease testing
- Recommend condoms with more reliable method (i.e., pills)
- Risk factors for early sexual activity:
  - Low socioeconomic status
  - Living in single parent home
  - Risk-taking behavior (smoking, alcohol, drugs)
  - Early or rapid pubertal development

SEXUAL ABUSE

- Perpetrators often male adult acquaintances
- Signs for suspicion:
  - Vaginal bleeding or trauma
  - Foreign body in vagina
  - Chronic vaginal or pelvic pain
  - Vulvovaginitis or sexually transmitted infection
  - Vague medical complaints (headache, painful defection)
  - Social or behavioral issues (anorexia, social problems, depression)
- Evaluation should include:
  - Examination of mouth, vagina, anus, inner thigh
  - Cultures for sexually transmitted infections
  - Forensic collection if within 72 hours of abuse
  - Semen can be detected with Wood lamp
  - Laboratory analysis for HIV, syphilis, hepatitis B, herpes simplex
- Must report suspected cases of sexual abuse
- Offer empiric treatment for gonorrhea, chlamydia, HIV

▶ DISORDERS OF PUBERTY

Precocious Puberty

- Signs of puberty before age 8 (variable between ethnic groups).
- If signs of advanced bone age present on radiography, treatment is with monthly gonadotropin injections to suppress puberty.

CENTRAL PRECOCIOUS PUBERTY

- *Gonadotropic dependent* (initiated by hypothalamic ovarian axis).
- Most common etiology is idiopathic.
- Other causes: Brain tumors, hydrocephalus, meningitis, encephalitis, brain abscess, head trauma, congenital adrenal hyperplasia.
- Diagnosis:
  - LH:FSH ratio >1, gonadotropins in pubertal range
  - Fasting 17-hydroxyprogesterone for congenital adrenal hyperplasia

PERIPHERAL PRECOCIOUS PUBERTY

- Gonadotropin independent (hypothalamic ovarian axis not activated).
- Causes include ovarian tumors, adrenal tumors and exogenous steroids.
- Diagnosis:
  - LH:FSH ratio <1, gonadotropins in prepubertal range
  - Ultrasound, CT, MRI to diagnose ovarian or adrenal tumor

INCOMPLETE PRECOCIOUS PUBERTY

- Premature thelarche—early breast development only.
- Premature adrenarche—isolated pubic or axillary hair.
- Vaginal bleeding only may be due to foreign object.
- Diagnosis:
    - LH:FSH <1, gonadotropins in prepubertal range
    - Elevated DHEA, testosterone with premature adrenarche

Delayed Puberty

- Absence of any secondary sexual characteristics by age 13.
- Constitutional delay is most common cause.

HYPERGONADOTROPIC HYPOGONADISM

- Ovarian failure (unresponsive ovary)
- Most common cause: Turner syndrome
- Other causes include:
    - Pure gonadal dysgenesis (Swyer syndrome, 46XY)
    - Mixed gonadal dysgenesis (45X, 46XY)
    - Chemotherapy, radiation therapy, autoimmune oophoritis

HYPOGONADOTROPIC HYPOGONADISM

- Failure of hypothalamus or pituitary.
- May be transient or permanent failure.
- Delay beyond age 15 unlikely to be constitutional.
- Differential diagnosis is Kallmann syndrome, anorexia, sports, pituitary tumor, idiopathic.

DIAGNOSIS

- Evaluation of thyroid, Tanner staging, vaginal smear, recto-abdominal exam
- Reduced sense of smell is hallmark of Kallmann syndrome
- Laboratory tests: CBC, thyroid tests, prolactin, gonadotropins (FSH, LH)
- Ultrasound to identify gonadal dysgenesis or lack of uterus
- Karyotype if evidence of primary hypogonadism
- MRI of head if neurologic symptoms present

▶ MENSTRUAL CYCLE

Menstrual Cycle Phases

FOLLICULAR PHASE

- See Figure 5–1 for changes during menstrual cycle.
- **Granulosa cells** produce estrogen and **theca cells** produce androgen.
- Antral or dominant follicle selected day 5–7.
- Estradiol results in negative feedback on FSH and positive feedback on LH.
- LH surge promotes continuation of meiosis in oocyte.

LUTEAL PHASE

- **Corpus luteum** is granulosa cells of follicle, which secrete progesterone. It regresses after 12–16 days unless pregnancy occurs.

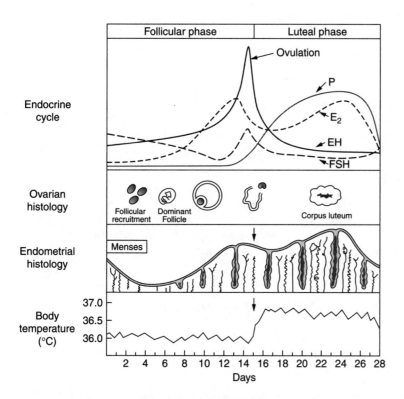

FIGURE 5-1. Endocrine, ovarian, endometrial, and basal body temperature changes and relations throughout the normal menstrual cycle.

(Adapted from Carr BR, Wilson JD. Disorders of the ovary and female reproductive tract. In: Kasper DL, Braunwald E, Fauci AS, Hauser SL, et al, eds. *Harrison's Principles of Internal Medicine.* 16th ed. New York, NY: McGraw-Hill, 2005: 2201, Fig. 326.4.)

Endometrial Changes

- **Decidua basalis:**
    - Deep layer which is source of regeneration after each menses.
    - Does not undergo significant change with cycle.
- **Decidua functionalis:**
    - Superficial layer which proliferates and sheds each cycle.
    - During proliferative phase estrogen stimulates simple columnar cells to change into pseudostratified pattern.
    - During secretory phase progesterone stimulates glycogen containing vacuole production by endometrial glands.
    - In absence of implantation, spiral artery vasospasm leads to decidua functionalis breakdown resulting in menses.

▶ DYSMENORRHEA

Definitions

- Primary dysmenorrhea:
    - Painful menses in absence of known pelvic pathology.
    - Related to arachidonic acid metabolites and prostaglandin production.
- Secondary dysmenorrhea:
    - Results from pelvic condition such as endometriosis, pelvic inflammatory disease, leiomyomata

RISK FACTORS

- Early menarche
- Long menstrual periods
- Smoking
- Alcohol
- Obesity
- Exacerbated by stress, caffeine, loss of sleep

DIAGNOSIS

- History and physical examination
- Cervical cultures to rule out infectious cause
- Pelvic ultrasound or sonohysterography to evaluate fibroids
- Laparoscopy to rule out endometriosis

TREATMENT

- Nonsteroidal anti-inflammatory agents (ibuprofen, mefenamic acid, ketoprofen)
- Hormonal contraceptives (oral, patch, ring)
- Exercise, dietary changes (low fat, vegetarian)
- Presacral neurectomy in extreme cases

▶ AMENORRHEA

Definition

- Primary amenorrhea:
  - No menses by age 16 with normal secondary sexual characteristics.
  - No menses by age 14 and absence of any secondary sexual characteristics.
- Secondary amenorrhea:
  - Absence of menses ≥6 months in woman who previously had menses.

ETIOLOGY

- Primary amenorrhea is usually the result of genetic or anatomic abnormality.
- Secondary amenorrhea is the most often caused by is pregnancy.

OVARIAN DISEASE (40–50%)

- **Gonadal agenesis:**
  - Significantly elevated FSH due to absence of ovarian response.
  - Causes include:
    - Turner syndrome (most common)
    - 46XX gonadal dysgenesis
    - 46XY gonadal dysgenesis (Swyer syndrome) is rare
  - 46XX and 46XY gonadal dysgenesis require gonadectomy.
- **PCOS:**
  - Second most common cause of secondary amenorrhea (after pregnancy)
  - May present as primary amenorrhea
  - Excess androgen mainly from ovary, but may come from adrenal gland

- Ovarian hyperthecosis:
  - Hyperandrogenism induces anovulation and endometrial atrophy
- **Premature ovarian failure:**
  - Cessation of menses <age 35
  - FSH > 40 mIU/mL
  - Causes may include:
    - Autoimmune dysfunction.
    - Genetic abnormalities.
    - Radiation or chemotherapy.
    - Gonadotropin resistance (savage syndrome) is rare.
  - If occurs <age 30, karyotype to rule out Turner syndrome or presence of Y chromatin material.

Gonadal dysgenesis is most common cause of primary amenorrhea. Pregnancy is most common cause of secondary amenorrhea.

HYPOTHALAMIC DYSFUNCTION (20–30%)

- **Chronic hypothalamic anovulation:**
  - LH and FSH are normal and lead to tonic estradiol levels.
  - Positive progestin challenge (response seen).
- **Functional hypothalamic amenorrhea:**
  - Decreased GnRH secretion leads to absent LH surge and anovulation.
  - Low LH/FSH ratio.
  - Usually no response to progestin challenge (low estradiol due to low FSH).
  - Caused by low body weight, stress, strenuous exercise, chronic illness.
- **Congenital GnRH deficiency:**
  - Hypogonadotropic hypogonadism
  - Low, apulsatile gonadotropin release
  - If anosmia present, consider Kallmann syndrome
  - Can be inherited, but 60% of cases sporadic
- **Brain diseases:**
  - Can result in decreased GnRH secretion
  - Neurological symptoms often present
  - Causes may include:
    - Infiltrative: Lymphoma, sarcoidosis
    - Tumors: Craniopharyngiomas
    - Injury: Trauma, hemorrhage, hydrocephalus
- **Drugs:**
  - Recreational, steroids, psychotropic

Chronic hypothalamic anovulation results in normal serum estradiol and has a positive response to progestin challenge. Functional hypothalamic amenorrhea results in decreased estradiol and no response to progestin challenge.

UTERINE OR VAGINAL ABNORMALITY

- Accounts for 20% primary and 5% secondary amenorrhea
- **Müllerian agenesis (Mayer-Rokitansky-Küster-Hauser syndrome):**
  - 46 XX.
  - Second most common cause of primary amenorrhea (second to gonadal dysgenesis).
  - Congenital absence of vagina. Normal hair pattern, normal testosterone.
  - Most have cervical and uterine agenesis, but 10% have functional endometrium.
  - No increased incidence of malignant tumors.
  - 25–50% have urinary tract abnormalities.
  - 10–15% have skeletal anomalies.
- **Androgen insensitivity** (previously testicular feminization):
  - 46XY, X-linked recessive disorder.

In patients with androgen insensitivity syndrome, gonadectomy should be performed after puberty because of risk of malignancy.

Presence of pubic and axillary hair helps differentiate müllerian agenesis from androgen insensitivity.

- Androgen receptor defect.
- Blind vagina, absent uterus, large breasts, parse sexual hair, normal or slightly elevated testosterone.
- Müllerian inhibiting factor produced by testes causes regression of müllerian structures.
- Commonly see breast development at puberty with pale areolae.
- Testes may be palpable in labia or inguinal area.
- Testes should be removed after puberty (5% incidence of malignancy).
- **5α-Reductase deficiency:**
  - 46XY
  - Female or ambiguous genitalia at birth.
  - Testosterone not converted to DHT, results in lack of external genitalia and prostate enlargement.
  - Virilization occurs at puberty due to increase in testosterone.
- **17α-Hydroxylase deficiency:**
  - Occurs in both 46XX and 46XY
  - Female or ambiguous genitalia with hypertension
  - Decreased cortisol. Increased ACTH, corticosterone, deoxycorticosterone
- **Asherman syndrome:**
  - Scarring of endometrial lining after postpartum hemorrhage or endometrial infection after instrumentation
- **Imperforate hymen:**
  - Cyclic pelvic pain and perirectal mass from blood sequestration in vagina
- **Transverse vaginal septum:**
  - Septum may occur anywhere between hymen and cervix (see vaginal defects on page 140).

PITUITARY DISEASE

- Accounts for 5% of primary and 20% of secondary amenorrhea
- **Hyperprolactinemia:**
  - Suppresses GnRH secretion
  - Presents similar to hypothalamic amenorrhea
  - Galactorrhea often present
- **Hypothyroidism:**
  - Thyrotropin releasing hormone stimulates prolactin secretion.
- **Empty sella syndrome:**
  - Enlarged sella turcica not entirely filled with pituitary tissue.
  - Causes include:
    - Surgically removed mass
    - Radiation
    - Infarction
- **Sheehan syndrome:**
  - Pituitary infarction after postpartum hemorrhage
- **Tumors:**
  - Nonlactotrophic adenomas
  - Infiltrative lesions

DIAGNOSIS

HISTORY AND PHYSICAL

- See Table 5–1 for causes of primary amenorrhea.
- Assess pubertal development. Short stature may suggest Turner syndrome.

TABLE 5–1. Causes of Primary Amenorrhea Based on Physical Exam

	BREASTS PRESENT	BREASTS ABSENT
Uterus present	▪ Outflow tract anomalies ▪ Hypothalamic causes ▪ Pituitary causes ▪ Ovarian causes	▪ Gonadal agenesis in 46XX ▪ Turner syndrome ▪ Disruption of hypothalamic axis
Uterus absent	▪ Müllerian agenesis ▪ Testicular feminization	▪ Gonadal agenesis in 46XY ▪ 17α-hydroxylase deficiency ▪ 5α-hydroxylase deficiency

- Headaches, visual changes, fatigue, polyuria, and polydipsia may indicate hypothalamic-pituitary disease.
- Galactorrhea may indicate pituitary disease.
- Signs of hyperandrogenism include hirsutism, acne, striae, acanthosis nigricans, vitiligo, and easy bruising.
- Medications which can cause amenorrhea are depo-Provera, depo-Lupron, danazol, high-dose progestins, metoclopramide, and antipsychotic drugs.
- Body dimensions and habitus:
  - BMI >30 kg/m^2 suggests PCOS.
  - BMI <18.5 kg/m^2 suggests functional hypothalamic amenorrhea.

DIAGNOSIS

- See Figure 5–2 for primary amenorrhea and Figure 5–3 for secondary amenorrhea.
  - Testosterone ↑ in 5α-reductase deficiency.
- FSH:
  - High in Turner syndrome or gonadal agenesis 46XX
  - Low or normal suggests hypothalamic-pituitary axis disorder
- Prolactin:
  - High prolactin may be transient. Check twice before cranial imaging
  - See pituitary causes of amenorrhea.
- If hypertension present, rule out 17α-hydroxylase deficiency:
  - Progesterone (↑)
  - Deoxycorticosterone (↑)
  - 17α-Hydroxyprogesterone (↓)
- High androgen:
  - May be PCOS or androgen-secreting tumor of ovary or adrenal gland.
  - Rapid onset of virilization more common with tumor.
  - 17-Hydroxyprogesterone and DHEA-S elevated in adrenal hyperplasia.
  - 24 Hour urinary free cortisol to evaluate Cushing syndrome.
- If history suspicious for Asherman syndrome, confirm diagnosis with hysterosalpingogram, hysteroscopy, or sonohysterogram.
- Progestin challenge:
  - Positive test (bleeding after withdrawal) sign of estrogen production
  - Negative test (no bleeding) consistent with hypothalamic dysfunction, outflow tract abnormality, Asherman syndrome

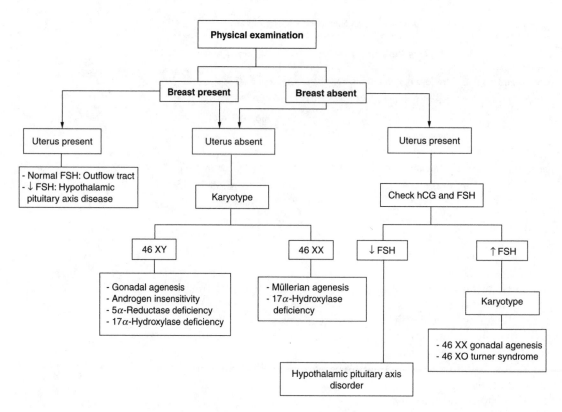

FIGURE 5–2. **Work up for primary amenorrhea.**

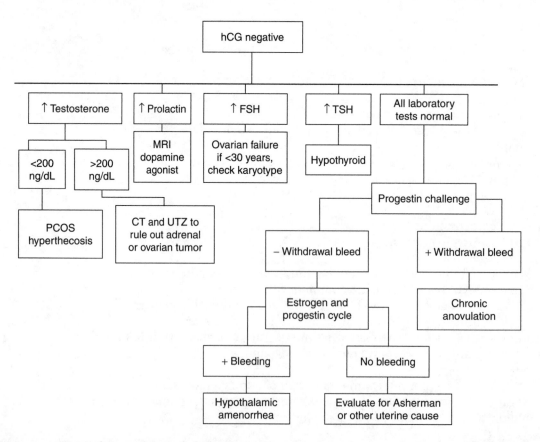

FIGURE 5–3. **Approach to management of secondary amenorrhea.**

TREATMENT

- **Hypothalamic dysfunction:**
  - Hormonal contraceptives help resume menses.
  - Athletic women should be counseled regarding adequate caloric intake and be started on hormonal contraceptives.
  - Women with eating disorders should be referred to nutritionist with multidisciplinary team.
- **Ovarian disease:**
  - Gonadal dysgenesis requires removal of ovaries or testes.
  - Counsel regarding hormone therapy. Benefits of osteoporosis prevention outweigh risks of myocardial infarction, stroke, and breast cancer.
  - PCOS treatment is hormonal cycling to prevent sequelae of prolonged unopposed estrogen or ovulation induction if pregnancy desired.
- **Anatomic causes:**
  - Imperforate hymen or transverse vaginal septum surgically corrected.
  - Müllerian agenesis treated with progressive dilation of pseudovagina or creation of neovagina with McIndoe procedure.
  - Asherman syndrome treated with hysteroscopy, lysis of adhesions. Pregnancy rates are 70–80% after treatment.
- **Pituitary disease:**
  - Hyperprolactinemia treated with dopamine agonists.
  - Hypothyroidism corrected with thyroid hormonal treatment.

Up to 70–80% of patients with Asherman syndrome achieve pregnancy after treatment.

▶ HYPERPROLACTINEMIA

Definition

- Prolactin levels ≥25 μg/L
- 50% with hyperprolactinemia have galactorrhea
- 20% with galactorrhea have hyperprolactinemia

CAUSES

- Pituitary hyperplasia (or idiopathic)
- Prolactinomas:
  - Microprolactinomas (<1 cm) or macroprolactinomas (≥1 cm)
  - Prolactin levels can be up to 1000 μg/L
- Hypothyroidism as elevated TRH stimulates prolactin release
- Drug intake:
  - Antidepressants, steroid hormones, antihypertensives, oral contraceptives
  - Prolactin levels usually between 25 μg/L and 100 μg/L
- Stress-induced prolactin rarely >40 μg/L
- Other causes:
  - Pregnancy
  - Trauma
  - Infection
  - Breast manipulation
  - Renal failure
  - Herpes zoster
  - PCOS

Clinical Manifestations

- Galactorrhea
- Ovulatory dysfunction with amenorrhea or oligomenorrhea

- Infertility
- Headaches and visual disturbances if prolactinoma present
- Androgen excess manifested by acne and hirsutism
- Osteopenia (due to decreased estradiol)

DIAGNOSIS

- hCG to exclude pregnancy
- Multiple measurements as prolactin released in pulsatile fashion
- Thyroid function tests (free thyroxine, TSH)
- MRI or CT, if thyroid function tests are normal
- Visual field testing if macroadenoma ≥1 cm

TREATMENT

- Based on symptoms, desire for fertility and tumor presence and size.
- Thyroid dysfunction should be corrected.
- Drug induced hyperprolactinemia should prompt discontinuation of medication.
- Prolactinoma treatment:
  - Dopamine agonists suppresses prolactin and cause tumor shrinkage:
    - Bromocriptine acts on dopamine D1 and D2 receptors.
    - Cabergoline is pure D2 receptor agonist.
    - Adverse effects: Nausea, lethargy, nasal congestion, dysphoria.
  - If dopamine agonist not used, estrogen replacement or contraception should be given to prevent bone loss.
  - Transsphenoidal hypophysectomy:
    - If unresponsive to medication or suprasellar extension of macroadenoma
    - High failure rate (70%)
- If pregnancy desired:
  - Treatment with dopamine agonist until prolactin levels normal.
  - Majority will resume ovulation when hyperprolactinemia corrected.
  - Once pregnancy established, medication should be:
    - Discontinued if microadenoma or functional hyperprolactinemia
    - Continued if macroadenomas (or discontinued and followed with visual field testing every 2 months)
  - Imaging studies not recommended during pregnancy unless symptomatic or abnormal visual field testing.

► PREMENSTRUAL DYSPHORIC DISORDER

Definition and Incidence

- Symptoms that significantly interfere with some aspect of life occurring strictly in luteal phase of menstrual cycle.
- 5–10% of reproductive age women.

RISK FACTORS

- Age >30
- Family history
- Affective disorder
- Not related to personality type, level of stress, culture, or socioeconomic status

TABLE 5-2. Diagnostic Criteria for Premenstrual Syndrome

At least one of the following affective and somatic symptoms during the 5 days before menses in all of three prior menstrual cycles

Affective	**Somatic**
■ Depression	■ Breast tenderness
■ Angry outbursts	■ Abdominal bloating
■ Irritability	■ Headache
■ Anxiety	■ Swelling of extremities
■ Confusion	
■ Social withdrawal	

ETIOLOGY

- Neurobiological vulnerability to fluctuation of sex steroids
- Common theory is serotonin dysregulation caused by sex steroid interaction:
  - Supported by success with selective serotonin reuptake inhibitors (SSRIs)

DIAGNOSIS

- See Tables 5–2 and 5–3 for diagnostic criteria of premenstrual syndrome and premenstrual dysphoric disorder.
- Based on 3–4 months of prospective symptom diaries (50% will have other pattern)
- Laboratory tests only if clinical suspicion of medical disorder (e.g., TSH)
- Differential diagnosis:
  - Psychiatric disorder: Depressive, panic, generalized anxiety disorder
  - Medical disorder: Migraines, irritable bowel syndrome, chronic fatigue, asthma, thyroid, adrenal disorders
  - Menopause

TABLE 5-3. Diagnostic Criteria for Premenstrual Dysphoric Disorder

- In most cycles during past year, ≥5 of the following usually present during last week of luteal phase, absent during week postmenses. At least one must be from items 1–4.
  1. Marked depressed mood, hopelessness, self-deprecating thoughts
  2. Marked anxiety, tension, feeling "keyed up" or "on edge"
  3. Persistent and marked anger, irritability, or increased interpersonal conflict
  4. Decreased interest in usual activities
  5. Lethargy, lack of energy, easy fatigability
  6. Marked change in appetite, overeating, or craving specific foods
  7. Hypersomnia or insomnia
  8. Subjective sense of being overwhelmed or out of control
  9. Other physical symptoms (breast tenderness, headaches, joint/muscle pain, bloating, weight gain)
- Disturbances interfere with work, school, social activities, and relationships.
- Must not be exacerbation of underlying disorder (major depressive disorder, panic disorder, dysthymia).

TREATMENT

- SSRIs should be considered for anyone with severe symptoms:
  - Fluoxetine (Prozac, Sarafem) in lower doses (20 mg/day) than for depression
  - Sertraline (Zoloft) late luteal phase dosing (14 days prior to menses)
- Oral contraceptive reduces symptoms
- Supportive therapy (reassurance, education, relaxation therapy)
- Aerobic exercise
- Dietary supplementation:
  - Calcium reduces symptoms after 2 months of use.
  - Primrose oil may be useful for breast tenderness.
  - Vitamin B_6 has limited benefit. Peripheral neuropathy possible if >100 mg/day.

▶ HIRSUTISM

Definition and Incidence

- Terminal, coarse hair in a male pattern (upper lip, chin, chest, back, abdomen)
- Affects 5–15% of women
- Sign of underlying androgen excess or hyperandrogenism

DIFFERENTIAL DIAGNOSIS

- Idiopathic hirsutism.
- PCOS is the most common etiology—see Polycystic Ovary Syndrome section.
- Congenital adrenal hyperplasia (nonclassical):
  - 21-Hydroxylase deficiency results in failure to metabolize 17-hydroxy-progesterone
  - Common in Hispanics and Ashkenazi Jews
  - Elevated 17-hydroxyprogesterone levels (>8 ng/mL)
  - ACTH stimulation may be done to confirm diagnosis
- Hyperandrogenic insulin resistance.
- Androgen-secreting tumors:
  - Virilization
  - Markedly elevated testosterone (>150 ng/dL)
  - May see elevated DHEA-S or androstenedione
- Androgenic drug intake.

TREATMENT

- Androgen suppression:
  - Oral contraceptive pills reduce circulating androgen levels by decreasing LH and increasing sex hormone-binding globulin (SHBG) levels.
  - GnRH agonists suppress LH secretion.
- Androgen receptor blockers:
  - Spironolactone, an aldosterone antagonist, binds to androgen receptor. Can combine with oral contraceptives. Side effects are hypotension and hyperkalemia (very rare).
  - Flutamide is nonsteroidal androgen receptor blocker. As effective as spironolactone. Potential hepatotoxicity requires liver function monitoring.

- 5α-Reductase inhibitor:
  - Finasteride inhibits conversion of testosterone to DHT.
- Mechanical control of hirsutism:
  - Hair elimination with shaving, chemical depilatories, electrolysis, laser.

▶ POLYCYSTIC OVARY SYNDROME

Definition

- Chronic anovulation and hyperandrogenism
- Affects 4–6% of reproductive age women

DIAGNOSTIC CRITERIA FOR PCOS

- See Table 5–4 for criteria for PCOS diagnosis

Pathophysiology

- Altered gonadotropin secretion:
  - Increased LH pulse frequency and amplitude:
    - Results in increased LH concentration
    - Correlates to increased pulse frequency of GnRH secretion
    - Results in excess ovarian androgen production
  - Elevated LH:FSH ratio often seen.
- Insulin resistance:
  - Insulin resistance with compensatory hyperinsulinemia stimulates theca cell androgen production in ovary.
  - 25–50% of women with PCOS are obese.
  - Insulin resistance suggested if:
    - ↑ fasting or serum insulin
    - Impaired glucose tolerance by 2-hour oral glucose tolerance test
    - Acanthosis nigricans
    - BMI >27 kg/m^2
    - Waist: hip ratio >0.85

DIAGNOSTIC TESTS

- Total and free stosterone:
  - Usually <150 ng/dL
  - Can be in normal or elevated range

TABLE 5–4. Criteria for Diagnosis of PCOS

1990 NICHD Criteria (requires all three):
- Chronic anovulation
- Clinical or biochemical evidence of hyperandrogenism
- Exclusion of other known etiologies

2003 Rotterdam Criteria (requires two of first three):
- Chronic oligomenorrhea or anovulation
- Clinical or biochemical evidence of hyperandrogenism
- Polycystic ovaries
- Exclusion of other known etiologies

- LH:
  - Confirm diagnosis, tends to be elevated
- FSH:
  - Confirm diagnosis, tends to be low or normal
- 17α-Hydroxyprogesterone:
  - Rule out nonclassical congenital adrenal hyperplasia
- 2-Hour glucose tolerance test and insulin:
  - Screen for diabetes
- Prolactin:
  - Rule out hyperprolactinemia
- TSH:
  - Rule out thyroid disease

MEDICAL CONSEQUENCES OF PCOS

- Three- to sevenfold increased risk of type 2 diabetes mellitus.
- Increased risk of cardiovascular disease because associated with dyslipidemia. Fasting lipid panel should be obtained.
- Increased risk of endometrial cancer, abnormal uterine bleeding, and infertility.

TREATMENT OF PCOS

- Diet modification, exercise, and weight loss:
  - Reduces insulin resistance.
  - Reduces hyperandrogenism.
  - Improves ovulation.
  - Decreases risk of cardiovascular disease and diabetes mellitus.
- Regulation of menstrual cycle:
  - Combination oral contraceptives are usual treatment.
  - Cyclic withdrawal bleeding reduces endometrial cancer risk.
- Ovulation induction:
  - Clomiphene citrate is first-line, increased risk of hyperstimulation.
  - Insulin-sensitizing agents (i.e., metformin) can be used with clomiphene in women with insulin resistance.
  - Gonadotropins used when clomiphene citrate unsuccessful.
- Antiandrogen agents:
  - Inhibit androgen action. Also useful for treatment of hirsutism.
  - Spironolactone is first-line. Flutamide and finasteride have similar efficacy in treating hirsutism (see Hirsutism section).
  - Spironolactone usually combined with oral contraceptives.
- GnRH agonists:
  - Most useful for severe ovarian androgen excess.
  - Suppresses pituitary secretion of LH.
  - Associated with hypoestrogenic state with potential for bone loss unless given with hormone add-back regimen.
- Surgical treatment:
  - Ovarian wedge resection rarely performed. Can induce long-term cyclic menstrual function.
  - Laparoscopic ovarian drilling with cautery or laser suggested for patients resistant to ovulation induction. Pregnancy rates equivalent to three cycles of gonadotropin treatment, but effects are temporary.
  - In women approaching menopause with severe hyperandrogenism, oophorectomy can be considered.

► INFERTILITY

Definitions

- Inability to conceive after 1 year of frequent unprotected intercourse
- Primary infertility—never having been able to conceive
- Secondary infertility—history of prior conception

CAUSES OF INFERTILITY

- Unexplained (28%):
    - Age, poor fertilization and implantation, poor embryo quality
- Male factor (23%):
    - Abnormal semen analysis, vas obstruction, varicocele
- Ovulatory dysfunction (18%):
    - PCOS, premature ovarian failure, hyperprolactinemia, hypothalamic-pituitary-ovarian axis
- Tubal factor (14%):
    - Hydrosalpinges, ligated tubes
- Peritoneal factor (9%):
    - Endometriosis, adhesions from surgery, infection, ruptured appendix
- Coital problems (5%)
- Cervical factor (3%)

Evaluation of Infertility

- Initial consultation should include history, physical exam, preconceptional counseling, and counseling on coital frequency and timing.

MEDICAL HISTORY

- Couple:
    - Contraception methods
    - Previous treatment
    - Past reproductive performance
    - Sexual dysfunction
    - Medications and allergies
    - Past illness and injury
    - Past surgery
    - Sexually transmitted diseases
    - Use of tobacco, alcohol, drugs
    - Family history of mental retardation or birth defects
    - Occupation
- Female partner:
    - Dysmenorrhea or dyspareunia
    - Abdominal or pelvic pain
    - History of galactorrhea, hirsutism, or thyroid disease
- Male partner:
    - Gonadal toxin exposure (e.g., heat)

PHYSICAL EXAM

- Female partner:
    - Signs of androgen excess
    - Breast secretion

- Weight and body mass index
- Thyroid enlargement
- Uterine size, shape, and position
- Cervical abnormality
- Abnormal vaginal secretions, screening with cervical cultures
- Abdominal or pelvic tenderness
- Adnexal/cul-de-sac tenderness or mass
- Signs of systemic disease
- Male partner:
  - Signs of gynecomastia or inadequate virilization
  - Testicular/scrotal abnormalities (size, symmetry, consistency, varicocele)
  - Abnormalities of penis
  - Abnormality or absence of vas deferens or epididymides
  - Signs of systemic disease

DIAGNOSTIC TESTS FOR FEMALE PARTNER

- **Ovulatory function:**
  - Basal body temperature (BBT):
    - Rises 1–3 days after midcycle LH surge. Has poor sensitivity.
  - Day 21 serum progesterone:
    - Values >3 ng/mL presumptive of ovulation.
  - Ovulation predictor kits:
    - Urinary LH provides indirect evidence of ovulation.
  - Endometrial biopsy:
    - Histologic evaluation to confirm ovulation.
    - Should not use for routine evaluation of infertility.
  - Transvaginal ultrasound:
    - Signs of presumptive ovulation are follicular growth, collapse of follicle, and fluid in cul-de-sac.
- **Ovarian reserve:**
  - Day 3 FSH and estradiol:
    - FSH levels >10 IU/L associated with decreased ovarian reserve.
  - Clomiphene citrate challenge test:
    - Administration of clomiphene citrate cycle days 5–9 and determination of estradiol on day 3 and FSH day 10.
- **Uterine cavity and fallopian tubes:**
  - Hysterosalpingogram:
    - Preferred method to evaluate tubal patency.
    - Evaluation of size and shape of uterine cavity.
    - Can delineate uterine anomalies, polyps, submucous myomas, synechia.
  - Ultrasonography:
    - Transvaginal or transabdominal to assess myomas or polyps.
  - Saline sonohysterogram:
    - Evaluation of size and shape of uterine cavity.
    - Very sensitive for polyps, submucous myomas, and synechia.
  - Hysteroscopy:
    - Definitive method of uterine cavity evaluation.
    - Usually for evaluation or treatment of abnormalities demonstrated by saline sonohysterogram or hysterosalpingogram.
  - Laparoscopy:
    - Direct visualization of pelvic structures.
    - Can evaluate tubal patency with chromotubation.

- Indicated if endometriosis or tubal disease suspected or if unexplained infertility.
- **Cervical mucus:**
  - Postcoital test:
    - Limited test with variable and subjective results.
    - Cervical mucus or sperm-mucus abnormalities are rarely main cause of infertility.
    - Current infertility treatments bypass unrecognized cervical factor.

DIAGNOSTIC TESTS FOR MALE PARTNER

- **Semen Analysis:**
  - Two analyses at least 2 weeks apart with abstinence 2–3 days prior.
  - Normal semen values found in Table 5–5.
  - Isolated loss of motility warrants evaluation with antisperm antibodies.
  - If volume <1mL, postejaculatory urinalysis excludes retrograde ejaculation.
  - >1 million leukocytes/mL in ejaculate suggests pyospermia. Should be evaluated for genital tract infection or inflammation.
- **Endocrine evaluation:**
  - If abnormal semen analysis, sexual dysfunction, or evidence of specific endocrine disease, consider FSH, LH, total and free testosterone, and prolactin.

TREATMENT OF FEMALE INFERTILITY

OVULATION INDUCTION AGENTS

- **Clomiphene citrate (Clomid) :**
  - Antiestrogen binds estrogen receptors in hypothalamus and pituitary, blocking negative feedback. Results in follicular growth.
  - Indicated for normogonadotropic oligo-ovulatory or anovulatory women (PCOS, luteal phase defect, unexplained infertility).
  - Response monitored with urinary LH or transvaginal ultrasound.
  - Addition of metformin for insulin-resistant women.
  - Addition of dexamethasone if elevated DHEA-S levels.
  - Tamoxifen, like clomiphene, with similar ovulation and pregnancy rates.

TABLE 5–5. Normal Semen Analysis Reference Values

CHARACTERISTIC	VALUE
Volume	≥2.0 mL
pH	>7.2
Sperm concentration	>20 million/mL
Sperm motility	>50%
Sperm morphology	≥30% normal (WHO criteria)
	≥14% normal (Kruger criteria)
White cell count	<1 million/mL

- Gonadotropins:
  - Indicated for anovulatory women with:
    - Normal gonadotropin levels who have failed clomiphene.
    - Low gonadotropin levels with hypopituitarism.
  - Risks are multiple gestations, ovarian hyperstimulation syndrome (OHSS).
- **Dopamine agonists:**
  - Bromocriptine or cabergoline suppress prolactin synthesis.
  - Treatment of choice for hyperprolactinemic anovulation.

IN VITRO FERTILIZATION

- Indications include:
  - Absent or blocked fallopian tubes
  - Pelvic disease such as endometriosis
  - Failed tuboplasty
  - Male factor infertility
  - Unexplained infertility
- Preimplantation genetic diagnosis (PGD):
  - Can detect genetic abnormalities
  - Offered to patients who are affected or carriers of a genetic disease

SURGICAL OPTIONS

- Hysteroscopic resection of endometrial polyps, submucous myomas, or minor intrauterine adhesions in absence of other fertility factors.
- Fimbriolysis, fimbrioplasty, laparoscopic adhesiolysis, or tubal reanastomosis can be considered if in vitro fertilization (IVF) not an option.
- Laparoscopic ovarian drilling (see section on PCOs)

TREATMENT OF MALE INFERTILITY

- Intrauterine insemination (IUI) :
  - May increase fecundity if decreased total motile sperm (<20 million).
  - Best on day after urinary LH surge or 36 hours after hCG administration.
- IVF with intracytoplasmic sperm injection (ICSI) :
  - Offered to patients with severe male factor infertility (<5 million motile sperm or <5% normal morphology) who have failed IUI

▶ MENOPAUSE

Physiology

- Onset genetically predetermined
- Environmental influences that predispose earlier menopause are smoking, surgery, baseline health conditions, steroid use
- Consists of decreased estrogen, sex hormone–binding globulin, estrogen-testosterone ratio
- Decreased inhibin and estrogen result in elevated FSH

SYMPTOMS

- Abnormal uterine bleeding common due to anovulation
- Hot flushes occur in 75–80% due to rapid decline in estrogen
- Frequency and severity of symptoms correlate with estrogen decline

- Anxiety, depression, irritability, and mood swings are common
- Increased tension headaches and decrease in migraines is seen

Physical Changes

OSTEOPOROSIS

- Estrogen inhibits bone resorption
- Hip fracture risk doubled for each standard deviation reduction in bone mass
- Most common fracture sites: Lumbar vertebrae, distal radius, femoral neck
- Risk factors are:
  - Chronic low calcium intake
  - Low body weight
  - Tobacco
  - Corticosteroid use
  - Heavy alcohol use
  - Sedentary or poor general health
  - Asian or Caucasian
- Screening should be done for:
  - All patients >65 years
  - One or more risk factors
  - Present with fracture(s)
- Diagnosis made with DEXA scan of hip and lumbar spine:
  - T-score is standard deviation below young adult mean
  - T-score ≤ -2.5 defines osteoporosis
  - T-score between -1 and -2.5 defines osteopenia

COLLAGEN LOSS AND ATROPHY

- Significant decline in collagen (2% per year for 10 years after menopause)
- Estrogen deficiency results in thin, pale vaginal mucosa
- Vaginal pH increases (usually >5)
- Increased vaginitis, pruritus, dyspareunia, urethritis, dysuria
- Weakened endopelvic fascia increases uterine prolapse, urinary incontinence

CORONARY ARTERY DISEASE

- Leading cause of death in women
- Lifetime risk of death in postmenopausal women 31%
- Increased risk due to:
  - Increased LDL
  - Increased triglycerides
  - Decreased HDL

LABORATORY ANALYSIS

- Usually unnecessary to perform laboratory analysis in woman >50
- Elevated FSH (≥ 20)
- TSH to rule out thyroid disease if symptoms suggestive

TREATMENT

OSTEOPOROSIS

- Bisphosphonates (alendronate, risedronate):
    - For prevention and treatment
    - Induces apoptosis of osteoclasts and decrease bone resorption
- Selective estrogen receptor modulator (raloxifene):
    - Prevents bone loss
    - No effect on breast or endometrial tissue
    - May increase hot flashes, decrease LDL
- Calcium supplementation (1000–1500 mg daily)
- Vitamin D (400 IU daily)
- Regular weight-bearing exercise
- Hormone therapy:
    - Not first-line treatment
    - Preventive and therapeutic if started for vasomotor symptoms

VASOMOTOR SYMPTOMS

- Hormone therapy reduces symptoms of hot flashes significantly (up to 90%)
- Must discuss risks and benefits:
    - Increased cardiovascular disease, breast cancer, stroke
    - Reduced risk of osteoporosis and colon cancer
- Clonidine patch or pill:
    - Nonhormonal treatment of hot flashes
    - Works on central nervous system to control vasomotor symptoms
- SSRIs may improve hot flashes
- Phytoestrogens and other alternative therapies:
    - Soy: Effectiveness unclear. Can potentially reduce hot flashes.
    - Black cohosh: No large, controlled studies have been conducted.
    - Topical or "natural" hormones: No formal studies done. No confirmation that topical estrogens do not stimulate endometrium.

VAGINAL ATROPHY

- Vaginal preparations useful for dryness and incontinence due to atrophy.
- Treatment options include vaginal cream, vaginal ring, oral, or patch.
- Systemic absorption with vaginal creams is one fourth that of same dose orally.

DEPRESSION AND MOOD CHANGES

- SSRIs often helpful
- Therapy and relaxation techniques should be offered

LIBIDO

- Vaginal estrogen can improve dryness and lubrication.
- Estrogen and testosterone pills available but effect still not well supported.
- Transdermal testosterone patch may help in surgical removal of ovaries but can increase cholesterol and risk of heart disease.

CHAPTER 6

Oncology

Malaika Amneus, MD
Linda A. Lewis, MD
Jeannine Rahimian, MD, MBA
Malini Anand, MD
Mor Tzadik, MD, MS

160

Genetics

- **Oncogenes** are autosomal dominant genes:
  - They contribute to aberrant cell proliferation and differentiation.
  - Alteration of one allele sufficient for cancer progression.
- **Tumor suppressor genes** are autosomal recessive genes which:
  - Encode DNA binding proteins
  - Function to prevent cell division or trigger cell death
  - Include p53, retinoblastoma (Rb), p16, BRCA, FHIT, neurofibromatosis (NF1), Wilms tumor gene (WT1)
- **DNA repair genes** are typically autosomal recessive genes which:
  - Encode protein products that repair or remove damaged DNA.
  - Defects cause diseases such as xeroderma pigmentosum, Bloom syndrome, Fanconi anemia, ataxia telangestasia, hereditary nonpolyposis colorectal cancer.
- **Aneuploidy** is the gain or loss of chromosome(s) during cell division. Over- or under expression of proteins contributes to cancer development.
- Phases of the **cell cycle**:
  - G1 phase: Enzyme and regulatory protein synthesis.
  - S phase: Nuclear DNA content copied.
  - G2 phase: RNA and protein synthesis and repair of errors in DNA replication.
  - M phase: Nuclear division.
  - After M phase, cells enter G1, G0 (resting phase), or undergo apoptosis.

Physiology

Chemotherapy and radiation therapy work on actively cycling cells. Cells in G0 (resting) phase are resistant. Goal is to balance treatment of tumor cells with harmful effects on normal cells (**therapeutic index**). Normal cells can often repair damage more effectively than neoplastic cells.

- Radiation therapy results in:
  - Apoptosis when DNA damage cannot be repaired.
  - Cell physiology changes: Edema, DNA fragmentation, bizarre nuclei, cell death.
  - Clinical effects: Diarrhea, tenesmus, hematochezia, dysuria, frequency, urgency.
  - Late effects: Hemorrhagic cystitis, reduced bladder capacity, proctitis, sigmoiditis, bowel obstruction, fistula, vaginal stenosis, radiation necrosis.
  - Second malignancies result from induced mutations. Most often leukemia, breast cancer.

Embryology and Anatomy

OVARY

- Primary oocytes arise from posterior wall of primitive gut, migrate into gonads.
- Ovaries descend into pelvis around 12 weeks gestation.
- Fixed by the suspensory ligament and mesovarium.
- Blood supply: Ovarian artery (anastomoses with uterine artery).
- Right ovarian vein drains into inferior vena cava, left vein into left renal vein.
- Innervated by hypogastric and ovarian plexuses.

FALLOPIAN TUBE

- Lies free in broad ligament
- Four parts: Infundibulum, fimbria, ampulla, isthmus
- Blood supply: Ovarian artery
- Innervated by hypogastric and ovarian plexuses

UTERUS

- Mullerian duct fuses with gubernaculum of Hunter to form uterine fundus.
- Fixed by levator ani muscles and broad, round, cardinal, and uterosacral ligaments.
- Blood supply: Uterine artery, ovarian artery.
- Venous drainage: Uterine and vaginal plexus.
- Innervated by hypogastric plexus (uterovaginal portion).

Pharmacology and Chemotherapy

- **Platinum compounds** incorporate a metallic element for cytotoxicity.
- **Antimicrotubule agents** stop cell cycle in metaphase.
- **Topoisomerase inhibitors** interfere with DNA topoisomerase enzymes.
- **Alkylating agents** cause DNA strand breaks which stop replication and transcription.
- See Table 6–1 for a review of chemotherapy side effects.
- Side effects should be treated as needed. Potential treatment options include:
  - Marrow suppression: Erythropoietin, G-CSF, GM-CSF, thrombopoietin
  - Nausea and vomiting: Selective serotonin receptor antagonists, corticosteroids, metoclopramide
  - Hemorrhagic cystitis: MESNA, hydration

TABLE 6–1. **Common Chemotherapeutic Agents and Their Toxicity**

CHEMOTHERAPY TYPES	AGENTS	MAJOR TOXICITIES
Platinum	Carboplatin	Myelosuppression
	Cisplatin	Nephrotoxicity, neurotoxicity, nausea
Antimicrotubule	Paclitaxel	Myelosuppression, alopecia, neurotoxicity
Taxanes	Taxotere	Myelosuppression, alopecia, peripheral neuropathy
Topoisomerase inhibitors	Topotecan	Myelosuppression, fatigue
	Etoposide	Myelosuppression, nausea, vomiting, leukemia
Alkylating	Cyclophosphamide	Myelosuppression, nausea, vomiting,
	Ifosfamide	Myelosuppression, nausea, vomiting, hemorrhagic cystitis, encephalopathy
Other	Doxorubicin	Myelosuppression, hand-foot syndrome, cardiotoxicity

- Peripheral neuropathy: Tricyclic antidepressants, vitamin B_6, Neurontin
- Renal toxicity: Hydration, amifostine

Microbiology and Immunology

- Cellular and humoral immune function worsens with cancer progression.
- Advanced stage disease associated with global immunosuppression.
- Chemotherapy and radiation therapy can suppress cellular immunity and result in myelosuppression.
- Immunosuppression increases risk of infection, poor wound healing.

▶ BREAST CANCER

Epidemiology

- Lifetime risk of invasive breast cancer is 1 in 8.
- Risk of dying from breast cancer is 1 in 28.
- Most common type of cancer and second most common cause of cancer death in women in the United States.
- Incidence highest in North America and Northern Europe, lowest in Asia and Africa, likely due to environmental rather than genetic factors.

RISK FACTORS

- **Gender:** 100 times more frequent in women than men.
- **Age:** Most significant risk factor.
- **Prolonged exposure to estrogen** (time and concentration):
  - Young age at menarche
  - Age of first full-term pregnancy >30
  - Late menopause
  - Nulliparity
  - Breast feeding *decreases* risk
- **Hormone replacement therapy:** Estrogen and progesterone, relative risk of 1.24 after 5 years. Unopposed estrogen not associated with increased risk.
- **Family history:** Only 10% of women diagnosed with breast cancer have a positive family history.
- **BRCA mutation carriers:**
  - BRCA1 (chromosome 17q21) and BRCA2 (chromosome 13q12.13) are autosomal dominant with high penetrance.
  - Lifetime risk of breast cancer with BRCA is 65–85%
  - Incidence of BRCA1 or BRCA2 in Ashkenazi Jewish population is 1 in 40.
  - Carriers should have breast exams and mammograms after age 25.
  - Prophylactic mastectomy decreases risk by 90%.
  - Bilateral salpingo-oophorectomy decreases risk of breast cancer by 40–50%.
- **Dietary factors:** Alcohol consumption and fat intake increase risk. One alcoholic drink per day increases risk slightly, 2–5 drinks per day increases risk more significantly.
- **History of breast conditions:**
  - Proliferative lesions without atypia (fibroadenoma, moderate to florid hyperplasia, sclerosing adenosis, and intraductal papilloma) have 1.3–2 fold increase in risk.
  - Atypical ductal hyperplasia increases risk four- to sixfold.

Breast cancer is the most common type of cancer and second most common cause of cancer death in women in the United States.

Age is the most significant risk factor for breast cancer. Only 10% of women diagnosed with breast cancer have a family history.

- Atypical lobular hyperplasia increases risk three- to fivefold.
- Lobular carcinoma in situ results in 1% per year risk of cancer.
- **Socioeconomic status:** Women of higher socioeconomic status are at greater risk. Thought to be due to factors such as parity and age at first birth.

DIAGNOSIS

MAMMOGRAPHY

- Used for screening of asymptomatic women.
- Efficacy depends on breast density (low density has high sensitivity).
- False negative rate: 10–15%.
- Suspicious findings:
  - Irregular shape
  - Spiculated borders
  - Pleomorphic calcifications that appear discontinuous, linear, and fine
- Benign microcalcifications: Large, coarse, vascular, or popcorn like.
- Breast Imaging Reporting and Data System (BI-RADS) classification system used for standardized mammogram reporting (see Table 6–2).
- Abnormal findings warrant further views, ultrasound, or biopsy.
- Distinct mass should always have biopsy regardless of mammogram findings.

ULTRASONOGRAPHY

- Can distinguish solid and cystic masses identified on clinical examination or mammogram.
- Used for ultrasound guided biopsy.
- Has a low specificity, therefore not good for screening.

FINE NEEDLE ASPIRATION

- Can differentiate between solid and cystic mass.
- Can treat and provide cytologic analysis for simple cysts.

TABLE 6–2. **American College of Radiology BI-RADS Categories**

CATEGORY	ASSESSMENT	RISK OF MALIGNANCY
0	Need additional imaging evaluation and/or prior mammograms for comparison	N/A
1	Negative	0
2	Benign findings	0
3	Probably benign findings: Initial short interval follow-up suggested	<2%
4	Suspicious abnormality; biopsy should be considered	2–75%
5	Highly suggestive of malignancy	75–95%

- Hematoma and inflammation can occur, so radiologic evaluation should always be done first.
- Disadvantage: Inability to distinguish between in situ and invasive cancer.
- False negative rate 3–35% (clinician experience). False positive rate is <1%.

CORE-NEEDLE BIOPSY

- Provides more definite diagnosis, less inadequate samples compared to FNA
- Performed with 14 gauge needle
- Most common biopsy technique
- Sensitivity and specificity as high as 97% and 99%
- If mass nonpalpable, should be done under image guidance

EXCISIONAL BIOPSY

- Incision and removal of entire mass under local anesthesia (outpatient procedure)
- Used for histologic diagnosis or complete excision of suspicious masses, calcifications, or core-biopsy proven tumor

Pathology

CARCINOMA IN SITU

- Confined to the basement membrane.
- Lobular carcinoma in situ (CIS) is more common in premenopausal women.
- Ductal CIS is more common in postmenopausal women. Leads to invasive cancer in 30–50% of women.

INVASIVE CARCINOMA

- Invades basement membrane and has risk of metastasis.
- Infiltrating ductal carcinoma is most common (70-80%).
- Infiltrating lobular carcinoma is second most common (10%).

PAGET DISEASE

- Resembles eczema.
- May be due to underlying malignancy extending into nipple/areola complex.
- Prognosis depends on underlying malignancy.

Staging

Clinical staging based on TNM system using tumor size, clinical assessment of axillary nodes, and presence or absence of metastases.

Prognostic Factors

- Axillary lymph node status is the most important prognostic factor.
- Number of positive nodes correlates with failure, metastases, survival.

Axillary lymph node status is the most important prognostic factor and correlates with survival rates.

- Better prognosis associated with:
  - Well-differentiated histology
  - Tumor size <1 cm
  - Hormone-positive receptors
  - Tumor types tubular, mucinous, medullary, adenoid cystic
- Poor prognosis associated with:
  - Micropapillary and inflammatory carcinomas
  - HER-2/neu overexpression

TREATMENT

- **Surgery** is performed for stage I and II disease. Options include:
  - Radical mastectomy: Removal of breast, pectoralis muscles, axillary contents. Significant morbidity without significant survival benefit so rarely performed.
  - Modified radical mastectomy: Same as radical except preservation of pectoralis major. No survival difference between radical and modified radical mastectomy.
  - Simple or total mastectomy: Removal of breast, nipple, areolar complex without pectoralis muscles or axillary lymph nodes.
  - Breast conserving therapy: Removal of tumor with 1–2 cm rim of normal tissue, usually followed by radiation.
- **Chemotherapy** used in:
  - Women <50 years regardless of hormone receptor status.
  - Most postmenopausal women with ER-negative tumors.
  - Most useful single agent is *doxorubicin*, but response rates higher with polyagent chemo (60–80%).
- **Radiation therapy**:
  - Used to treat subclinical disease and minimize recurrence.
  - High failure rate if used without tumor excision.
  - Ipsilateral whole-breast radiation is used in breast-conserving therapy.
- **Hormonal treatment** directed at cancer cells with estrogen or progesterone receptors:
  - Tamoxifen, an estrogen-receptor antagonist, reduces annual recurrence by 50% and annual odds of death by 25% when taken for 5 years.
  - In postmenopausal women, estrogen production inhibited by aromatase inhibitors (anastrozole, letrozole, exemestane).
  - In premenopausal women, ovarian estrogen inhibited by surgical or radiation castration, or LH-releasing analogs (leuprolide, goserelin).

Pregnancy and Breast Cancer

- **Incidence** of 1 in 3000 pregnancies. Second most common malignancy in pregnancy (after cervical cancer).
- **Survival rates** equivalent to nonpregnant women when matched by the stage of disease. Diagnosis limited by physiologic changes in breast that may delay diagnosis or limit the utility of mammogram.
- **Treatment recommendations:**
  - Local disease diagnosed in first or second trimesters should be treated with definitive surgery and radiation. Adjuvant chemotherapy can be given after the first trimester.
  - Local disease diagnosed in third trimester may be excised. Patient can have delivery followed by usual treatment for the given stage.

- Diagnosis in postpartum: Lactation should be suppressed, cancer treated definitively.
- Advanced cancer may be treated palliatively with or without continuation of pregnancy, depending on wishes of the mother.

▶ OVARIAN CANCER

- Lifetime risk is 1–2%.
- Risk factors: Age >60, BRCA carrier, family history of ovarian or breast cancer, infertility, low parity, high fat diet, personal history of breast or colon cancer.
- Oral contraceptives are protective:
  - Relative risk 0.7 after 2 years and 0.5 after ≥5 years.
  - Risk reduction persists after discontinuation.
  - Risk reduction may be seen in those with familial syndromes.
- Lifetime risk reduced in patients with:
  - Tubal sterilization
  - Hysterectomy
  - Breast feeding

Survival rates are equivalent when pregnant and nonpregnant women with breast cancer are matched by the stage of disease.

Screening

- No effective method of screening general population.
- CA125 ineffective because of high false-positive and false-negative rates.
- Transvaginal ultrasound has high false-positive rate.

Familial Syndromes

- >90% of ovarian cancer cases are sporadic.
- 5–10% of ovarian cancer associated with germline mutation. Usually have autosomal dominant transmission and early onset cancer (~40 years).
- Women with germline mutation should be offered prophylactic bilateral salpingo-oophorectomy after childbearing is complete.
- **BRCA1/BRCA2:**
  - Tumor suppressor gene mutations
  - Common in Ashkenazi Jewish population
  - Lifetime risk of ovarian cancer: BRCA1: 25–55%, BRCA2: 15–25%
- **Hereditary nonpolyposis colorectal cancer syndrome (Lynch II):**
  - Increased cancer of colon, breast, ovary, endometrium
  - Risk of ovarian cancer increased by 3.5 fold

Oral contraceptives reduce lifetime risk of ovarian cancer. Risk reduction may persist years after discontinuation and may be seen in those with familial hereditary syndrome.

DIAGNOSIS

- Symptoms: Increased abdominal size, bloating, fatigue, abdominal pain, inability to eat, urinary frequency, constipation
- Ultrasound findings: Solid components, septations, presence of flow in solid component, ascites, peritoneal masses, enlarged nodes, matted bowel

Staging

Should include TAH, BSO, peritoneal washings, infracolic omentectomy, pelvic and periaortic lymph node sampling, biopsies of diaphragm, and suspicious lesions

Women with germline mutation should be offered a prophylactic bilateral salpingo-oophorectomy after childbearing is complete.

Histology

EPITHELIAL OVARIAN CANCER

- Originates from coelomic epithelium.
- Accounts for 85–90% of ovarian cancer with distribution of:
  - Serous 40–50%
  - Endometrioid 15%
  - Mucinous 12–15%
  - Clear cell 5–10%
- CA-125 is an ovarian cell surface protein expressed in 80% of nonmucinous epithelial ovarian cancers. Can be elevated with pancreatitis, colon cancer, tuberculosis, pregnancy, pelvic inflammatory disease, fibroids, benign ovarian tumors.

PRIMARY PERITONEAL CANCER

- Difficult to distinguish from epithelial ovarian cancer.
- Extraovarian involvement must be greater than ovarian involvement.
- Requires serous histology for diagnosis.
- Diagnosis and workup similar to epithelial ovarian cancer.

GERM CELL TUMORS

- Originates from primordial germ cells.
- Accounts for 10% of ovarian cancers and 20% of all ovarian tumors.
- Most common in first two decades of life (10–30 years).
- Often have enzymatic activity (hCG, AFP, LDH). See Table 6–3 for markers.

Dysgerminoma is the most common malignant germ cell tumor:

- Bilateral in 10–15% so contralateral ovary should be biopsied.
- Gross appearance lobulated, firm, and yellow tan.
- Histology is undifferentiated germ cells.
- Often contains syncytiotrophoblastic giant cells.
- Produce alkaline phosphatase and LDH.

Endodermal sinus (Yolk sac) tumor is the most aggressive germ cell tumor:

- Derived from the primitive yolk sac.
- Median age 18 years.

TABLE 6–3. Markers for Germ Cell Tumors

TUMOR	AFP	HCG	LDH
Dysgerminoma	–	+/–	+
Embryonal carcinoma	+/–	+/–	–
Immature teratoma	–	–	–
Choriocarcinoma	–	+	
Endodermal sinus	+	–	–

- **Schiller-Duval bodies** and tubules lined with flattened cuboidal cells.
- Treatment is unilateral salpingo-oophorectomy and chemotherapy (BEP).

Embryonal carcinoma:

- Multinucleated giant cells resembling syncytial cells scattered throughout.
- Mean age 15 years.
- May produce estrogen, androgens, or AFP.
- 50% have hormonal abnormality (precocious puberty, irregular bleeding, amenorrhea).
- Pregnancy test positive (hCG).

Choriocarcinoma can be gestational or nongestational:

- Presence of paternal DNA confirms gestational.
- Very early hematogenous spread to placenta, lung, brain.
- Most common symptom is abnormal uterine bleeding.
- Associated with precocious puberty (due to hCG).

Teratoma contains fetal tissue from all germ layers and can be benign or malignant:

- Mature cystic (benign):
    - Most common germ cell tumor.
    - Accounts for 95% of teratomas.
    - Struma ovarii has thyroid tissue and can result in clinical hyperthyroidism.
- Immature solid (malignant):
    - Contain immature neural elements
    - Common in first two decades of life

Mature cystic teratomas are the most common germ cell tumor. Dysgerminomas are the most common malignant germ cell tumor.

STROMAL TUMORS

- Originates from mesenchymal tissue of the ovary.
- Accounts for 5% of ovarian cancer.
- Types include granulosa cell (>90) and Sertoli-Leydig (<10%).

Granulosa cell tumors:

- Most common in first four decades of life
- Bilateral in 5%
- Characterized by **Call-Exner bodies** (coffee bean nuclei)
- Theca cells, if present, produce **estrogen**. Results in precocious puberty, metrorrhagia, postmenopausal bleeding, endometrial hyperplasia (25–50%), endometrial cancer (5–10%)
- Malignant and late recurrences common
- Produces **inhibin** which can be used as a marker

Sertoli-Leydig tumors account for <1% of ovarian cancers:

- Rarely bilateral (<1%).
- Produces **testosterone**. Masculinizing features (amenorrhea, breast atrophy, acne, hirsutism) present in 40–80% of patients.
- Malignant potential related to degree of differentiation.

Endometrial hyperplasia and cancer is detected in 25–50% and 5–10% of patients with granulosa cell tumors.

LOW MALIGNANT POTENTIAL (BORDERLINE)

- 10% of malignant ovarian tumors
- Frequent in premenopausal women between 30 and 50 years

- 90% diagnosed in Stage I
- CA125 elevated in <25% patients

Histology

- Serous tumors are the most common and often bilateral (25–50%).
- Tumors associated with pseudomyxoma peritonei are often of appendiceal origin.
- Endometrioid, clear cell, transitional cell are rare and usually unilateral.

DIAGNOSIS

- Usually asymptomatic but some are present with a pelvic mass.
- Requires atypical nuclear atypia, increased mitotic activity, epithelial proliferation without stromal invasion.
- Frozen section used for diagnosis but ~20% found to be invasive at final review. Factors reducing reliability of frozen section are large tumor size and mucinous histology (more histologic variation).
- Staging not routinely performed, but useful if invasive cancer on final pathology.

SARCOMA

Rare and aggressive. Symptoms and diagnosis similar to epithelial ovarian carcinoma.

METASTATIC TUMOR

Most commonly from the gastrointestinal tract (Krukenberg tumor), breast, endometrium, lymphoma.

TREATMENT AND SURVIVAL

EPITHELIAL OVARIAN CANCER

- **Optimal cytoreduction** is excision of all tumor >1 cm. Improves chemotherapy response rate and overall survival.
- **Interval cytoreductive surgery** done after short cycle of chemotherapy and followed by chemotherapy has not been shown to have a survival benefit.
- Of the 50% cases in clinical remission after treatment, 50% have residual disease at **second look laparotomy**. Second look is not standard of care and does not affect outcome in clinically disease-free patients.
- About 75% respond to chemotherapy, which is used if:
  - Clear cell histology
  - Stages IB to IV
  - Grade 2–3
- **Follow-up** surveillance is with physical exam, CA125, annual pap smears. No proven benefit of routine CT scans.
- **5-year survival:**
  - Stage I: 74–93%
  - Stage II: 51–70%
  - Stage III: 23–40%
  - Stage IV: 10–25%

PRIMARY PERITONEAL CANCER

Treated like ovarian cancer with similar response rates.

GERM CELL TUMORS

- Patients who desire fertility: Unilateral salpingo-oophorectomy, washings, omentectomy, biopsies of pelvic and para-aortic lymph nodes and peritoneum.
- Chemotherapy required unless Stage IA, grade 1 dysgerminoma or Stage I, grade 1 immature teratoma.
- Long-term survival is 90–100% for dysgerminoma, 73–80% for immature teratoma, and 60–70% for endodermal sinus tumor.

STROMAL TUMORS

- Unilateral salpingo-oophorectomy with inspection of contralateral ovary.
- Chemotherapy is used for recurrent or metastatic disease.
- Granulosa cell tumor survival is 75–90% at 10 years.
- Sertoli-Leydig survival is 70–90% at 5 years.

LOW MALIGNANT POTENTIAL (BORDERLINE)

- Unilateral salpingo-oophorectomy and staging if fertility desired.
- TAH, BSO, omentectomy, staging if fertility not desired or if advanced disease.
- With mucinous histology: Appendectomy and abdominal exploration required.
- Chemotherapy is controversial. No survival benefit unless invasive implants present.
- Survival:
    - At 7 years: 99% if Stage I, 95% if Stage II
    - At 18 years: 8% recurrence, usually is confined to ovaries

SARCOMA

Treatment is cytoreductive surgery and platinum-based chemotherapy.

▶ CERVICAL NEOPLASIA

Epidemiology

- Incidence and mortality has declined 75% in the last 50 years in developed countries.
- One of the leading causes of cancer-related mortality in women worldwide.
- Incidence is twofold greater in African Americans than Caucasians.

RISK FACTORS

- Sexual activity started at early age
- Multiple sexual partners
- Smoking (relative risk ~two- to threefold)

Cervical cancer is one of the leading causes of cancer deaths in women worldwide.

- Human immunodeficiency virus (HIV) (cervical cancer is an AIDS-defining illness)
- Immunosuppressed, poor diet
- Low socioeconomic status
- Oral contraceptive use (more associated with adenocarcinoma)

Human Papilloma Virus (HPV)

- Present in 99% of invasive squamous cell cancers.
- Central causative agent but other factors promote or prevent carcinogenesis.
- High risk HPV types are: 16, 18, 31, 35, and 45.
- Oncogenes *E6* and *E7* inactivate tumor suppressor genes p53 and Rb, respectively.

DIAGNOSIS

- Most patients are asymptomatic and diagnosed with cytology screening.
- Symptoms: Abnormal or postcoital bleeding, watery or foul-smelling discharge. Diagnosis based on cervical biopsy of abnormal lesion or colposcopy directed.
- Diagnostic conization necessary if biopsy normal with abnormal cytology.
- Conization required for diagnosis of microinvasive disease and staging.
- Differential diagnosis: Nabothian cysts, glandular hyperplasia, endometriosis, mesonephric remnants.

Invasive cervical cancer is an AIDS-defining illness.

Pathology

Squamous cell carcinoma accounts for 80–90% of cervical cancers. Other types include:

- Adenocarcinoma (mucinous, clear cell, endometrioid, serous, mesonephric)
- Adenosquamous
- Other (glassy-cell, adenoid cystic, adenoid basal, neuroendocrine)

Staging

Cervical cancer staging based on **clinical evaluation.** The following are **allowed:**

- Examination of tumor and nodes
- Colposcopy
- Endocervical curettage
- Conization
- Hysteroscopy
- Cystoscopy
- Proctoscopy
- Intravenous pyelogram (IVP)
- X-ray of lungs and skeleton

Cervical cancer staging is based on clinical evaluation, not surgicopathologic findings.

Although not useful for FIGO staging, CT, MRI, and PET scans may be useful in treatment planning.

TREATMENT

- Options include surgical or radiation treatment. See Table 6–4 for treatment options by stage of cervical cancer.

TABLE 6–4. **Treatment of Cervical Cancer by FIGO Stage**

STAGE	TREATMENT
0 or IA1	Conservative with conization or simple hysterectomy
IA2	Radical hysterectomy
IA2, IB, or IIA	Radical hysterectomy with lymphadenectomy or radiation with concurrent low-dose cisplatin sensitization
IIB or greater	Radiation with concurrent low-dose cisplatin sensitization

- Benefits of surgical management:
  - More functional vaginal (length and lubrication reduced with radiation)
  - Possible preservation of ovarian function
  - Opportunity for abdominal exploration
  - Better pathologic information for treatment decisions
- Benefits of radiation therapy:
  - Avoids surgical morbidity and mortality
  - No risk of blood loss
- **Simple hysterectomy** (type I):
  - Removal of uterus and cervix
  - Ureters not disturbed
- **Modified radical hysterectomy** (type II)
  - Removal of uterus, cervix, upper portion of vagina
  - Distal half of uterosacral ligaments ligated
  - Uterine artery ligated medial to ureter
- **Radical hysterectomy** (type III):
  - Removal of uterus, cervix, upper third of vagina
  - Parametrial tissue to pelvic wall
  - Uterosacral ligaments ligated at origin
  - Uterine artery ligated lateral to ureter
- **Pelvic exenteration** considered only for patients with local pelvic recurrence.

SURVIVAL

Table 6–5 shows the survival rates of cervical cancer by FIGO stage.

TABLE 6–5. **Survival and Recurrence Rates of Cervical Cancer**

STAGE	5-YEAR SURVIVAL
I	82–85%
II	61–66%
III	37–39%
IV	11–12%

ONCOLOGY

TABLE 6–6. Treatment Options by Gestational Age and Stage of Cervical Cancer

STAGE	GESTATIONAL AGE <24 WEEKS	GESTATIONAL AGE ≥ 24 WEEKS
IA	Conization or hysterectomy	Cesarean at term with conization or hysterectomy
–IIA	Radical hysterectomy or radiation therapy	Cesarean at term with either radical hysterectomy or radiation therapy
IIB–IIIB	Radiation therapy	Cesarean at term with radiation therapy

Pregnancy and Cervical Cancer

One in 10,000 women with cervical cancer is pregnant. Pregnancy does not promote or accelerate the growth of cervical cancer. See Table 6–6 for treatment options.

▶ ENDOMETRIAL CANCER

- See Table 6–7 for comparison of types of endometrial cancer.
- Fourth most common cancer in women worldwide (after breast, lung, colon).
- Average age at diagnosis is 60 years.
- Most cases are type I and result from hyperestrogenism and hyperplasia.

RISK FACTORS

- Nulliparity, obesity, infertility, anovulatory cycles, early menarche, late menopause, unopposed estrogen, diabetes.
- Tamoxifen increases risk by two- to threefold.
- Family history of hereditary nonpolyposis colorectal cancer (HNPCC)
- Protective agents: Oral contraceptives, smoking.

TABLE 6–7. Characteristics of Endometrial Carcinoma Types

TYPE I	TYPE II
- Associated hyperestrogenism	- Not related to hyperestrogenism
- Associated with hyperplasia	- usually atrophic endometrium
- Patients usually young, perimenopausal	- Patients 5–10 years older at presentation
- Estrogen and progesterone receptors common	- Estrogen and progesterone receptors uncommon
- Usually endometrioid and mucinous subtypes	- Usually serous or clear cell subtypes
- More favorable prognosis	- More aggressive, poor prognosis

Screening

- No accepted method of screening asymptomatic population.
- If family history of HNPCC: Annual endometrial biopsy (EMB) screening >35 years.
- Tamoxifen users receive no benefit from screening.

DIAGNOSIS

- Symptoms: Intermenstrual spotting, menorrhagia, postmenopausal bleeding. Causes of postmenopausal bleeding include:
  - Endometrial atrophy (60–80%)
  - Estrogen replacement therapy (15–25%)
  - Endometrial polyp (2–12%)
  - Endometrial hyperplasia (5–10%)
  - Endometrial cancer (10%)
- Physical exam usually without significant findings.
- Ultrasound can be useful. Endometrial lining <5 mm in postmenopausal woman with bleeding has good negative predictive value.
- Diagnosis based on EMB or dilation and curettage (D&C)
- Hysteroscopy more accurate than EMB or D&C for diagnosis of polyps or myomas.

Histology

ENDOMETRIAL HYPERPLASIA

- Hyperplasia is the proliferation of endometrial glands with development of:
  - Irregular size and shape of glands
  - An increase in the gland/stromal ratio
  - Classified as simple or complex (based on glandular and stromal architecture) and with atypia or without atypia (based on the presence or absence of nuclear atypia).
- Rates of progression from hyperplasia to carcinoma are:
  - 1% of simple hyperplasia without atypia
  - 3% of complex hyperplasia without atypia
  - 8% of simple hyperplasia with atypia
  - 29% of complex hyperplasia with atypia

ENDOMETRIAL CARCINOMA

- Endometrioid: Most common (80%) and best prognosis.
- Others: Mucinous (5%), papillary serous (3–4%), adenosquamous (15%), and clear cell (<5%) tend to be more aggressive and carry a worse prognosis.

SARCOMAS

Sarcomas of the uterus represent 3–5% tumors and include the following:

- Stromal sarcomas (i.e., leiomyosarcoma)
- Mixed homologous (i.e., carcinosarcoma)
- Mixed heterologous (i.e., mixed müllerian tumor)

ONCOLOGY

- Rare types: Angiosarcoma, fibrosarcoma, rhabdomyosarcoma, chondrosarcoma, osteosarcoma, liposarcoma

TREATMENT

ENDOMETRIAL HYPERPLASIA

Medical treatment used when future fertility is desired. Treatment options include:

- Oral contraceptives (if no atypia)
- Progestin (medroxyprogesterone acetate, Megace, norethindrone)
- Gonadotropin releasing hormone analogs
- Ovulation induction agents
- Levonorgestrel containing IUD

Continuous regimens preferred for postmenopausal women or if with atypia. Treatment should be continued for 3–6 months and then repeat EMB done.

Surgery (i.e., hysterectomy) is recommended for complex hyperplasia with atypia if no desire for fertility as there is a high rate of coexisting endometrial carcinoma (~25%). Surgery is also considered if medical treatment contraindicated, failed, or declined.

ENDOMETRIAL CARCINOMA

- Treatment is surgical:
  - TAH, BSO, with staging procedure.
  - Cystoscopy or sigmoidoscopy if bladder or rectal involvement is suspected.
- Radiation therapy recommended if at high risk of recurrence or as alternative to surgery in poor surgical candidates.
- Hormonal therapy with progestins is often used for recurrent endometrioid tumors.
- Chemotherapy is controversial and generally reserved for palliative treatment.

SURVIVAL

Survival rates are approximately:

- Stage I: 87%
- Stage II: 76%
- Stage III: 51%
- Stage IV: 19%

Prognostic factors are histopathology, degree of differentiation, myometrial invasion, lymph vascular space invasion, tumor size, hormone-receptor status, peritoneal cytology, lymph node metastasis.

▶ VULVAR CARCINOMA

- Vulvar carcinoma accounts for 3–5% of gynecologic malignancies.
- Incidence increases with age.
- Squamous cell carcinoma is the most common type (90% of cases).

RISK FACTORS

- Sexual activity
- Genital condyloma or HPV
- Smoking
- Chronic vulvar conditions (e.g., lichen sclerosis)
- HIV (fourfold increase)

DIAGNOSIS

- Symptoms include pruritus, burning, edema, pain, mass, bleeding, and urinary symptoms.
- Lesions may be raised or flat, with or without pigmentation.
- Erythema, hyperkeratosis, ulceration, inguinal lymphadenopathy may be present.
- Acetic acid may enhance hyperkeratotic and condylomatous areas on vulva.
- Differential diagnosis:
  - Pigmented lesions: Vulvar intraepithelial neoplasia (VIN), benign nevi, lichen sclerosis, vulvar cancer
  - Erythematous lesions: VIN, inflammatory dermatitis, Paget's disease, vulvar cancer
- Punch biopsy preferred to minimize crush artifact.

Histology

VULVAR INTRAEPITHELIAL NEOPLASIA (VIN)

- High-grade VIN is a preinvasive lesion involving dysplastic squamous cells.
- **Basaloid type** is usually found in older women and is not associated with HPV. Often present in areas of atrophy (e.g., lichen sclerosis).
- **Bowenoid type** usually found in younger women and associated with HPV. Demonstrates multinucleation, koilocytosis.

VULVAR CARCINOMA

- **Squamous cell carcinoma** is the most common type of vulvar carcinoma (90%).
- **Melanoma** is second most common type. Usually seen in postmenopausal (mean age 60). Typically pigmented. Often on clitoris or labia minora.
- **Verrucous carcinoma**, a variant of squamous cell, is locally destructive, but rarely metastasizes. Typically cauliflower like in appearance.
- **Bartholin gland carcinoma** is the most common adenocarcinoma on vulva. Usually adenocarcinoma, but may be squamous cell or adenoid cystic. Occurs at ~age 40.
- **Paget disease** is an adenocarcinoma, located on hair-bearing areas of labia. Often associated with adenocarcinoma of skin, adnexa, or Bartholin gland. May be related to more distant carcinomas (e.g., breast, gastrointestinal, urinary tract).
- **Basal cell** carcinoma is described as "rodent ulcer" with pearly, rolled edges and central ulceration. Locally invasive, but rarely metastasize. Typically found in Caucasians, >70 years.

- **Sarcoma is** usually on labia majora and is very rare. Most common is leiomyosarcoma.

TREATMENT

VULVAR INTRAEPITHELIAL NEOPLASIA (VIN)

- **Ablation (CO_2 laser)** is effective for lesions on areas without hair, but no specimen is available for pathologic review.
- **Surgical excision** via local excision or partial superficial vulvectomy. Re-excision may be necessary.
- **Topical medications** such as imiquimod, 5-fluorouracil, bleomycin, or dinitrochlorobenzene are generally painful and results are inconsistent.

VULVAR CARCINOMA

Surgery is mainstay of therapy. Options include:

- Radical local excision or radical vulvectomy. Margins should be ≥1 cm.
- Inguinal femoral lymphadenectomy if ≥1 mm stromal invasion:
    - Lateral lesions: Ipsilateral lymphadenectomy
    - Midline or central lesions: Bilateral lymphadenectomy
- Exenteration may be necessary for large lesions that have invaded adjacent organs.

    Radiation either pre- or postoperative may be appropriate in some patients.
    Chemotherapy combined with radiation often used in advanced cases. Usually 5-fluorouracil and cisplatin.

SURVIVAL AND PROGNOSIS

5 year survival rates are:

- Stage I: 90%
- Stage II: 77%
- Stage III: 51%
- Stage IV: 18%

    Prognosis dependent on lymph node status:

- Number of nodes involved
- Size of nodes
- Whether node capsule intact

    Follow-up is with careful physical examination:

- Every 3 months for 1st year.
- Every 4 months for 2nd year.
- Every 6 months, 3rd through 5th years

► VAGINAL NEOPLASIA

- The majority of cancers in the vagina are metastatic.
- Primary vaginal cancer accounts for only 1–2% of gynecologic cancers.

- History of cervical cancer or carcinoma in situ strongly linked to vaginal cancer.

RISK FACTORS

- HPV, smoking, previous abnormal cervical or vaginal cytology, ≥5 lifetime partners.

DIAGNOSIS

- Symptoms may include vaginal bleeding (especially postcoital) and vaginal discharge, or no symptoms.
- Thickening, irregularity, or discoloration of vaginal wall.
- Application of dilute acetic acid may assist in visualization.
- Colposcopy with liberal biopsies should be performed if suspicious.
- CT of abdomen and pelvis and CXR if suspicious for metastatic disease.
- Cystoscopy and proctoscopy if suspicious of bladder and rectal invasion.

Histology

VAGINAL INTRAEPITHELIAL NEOPLASIA (VAIN)

- Associated with HPV
- Rare progression to vaginal carcinoma
- Usually occurs on posterior wall in upper third of vagina

VAGINAL CARCINOMA

- **Squamous cell carcinoma** is most common type. May present with nodules, induration, ulcers, or exophytic mass. Usually on posterior wall of upper third of vagina.
- **Adenocarcinoma (clear cell)** has polypoid appearance. Common in anterior upper third of vagina of women with in utero DES exposure (median age 19).
- **Sarcoma,** most commonly known as embryonal rhabdomyosarcoma (sarcoma botryoides), is a soft, edematous collection of nodules that fills vagina and protrudes from introitus. Most common in infants or young children.
- **Melanoma** usually presents as blue, black, or brown discoloration, mass, or ulcer. Nonpigmented lesions can also occur. Often in distal third of vagina.
- **Verrucous carcinoma** a variant of squamous cell type, presents as large, soft, cauliflower-like mass. Associated with HPV 6.

TREATMENT AND SURVIVAL

VAGINAL INTRAEPITHELIAL NEOPLASIA

- **Topical estrogen** used in postmenopausal women with vaginal intraepithelial neoplasia (VAIN), which is thought to be due to vaginal atrophy rather than neoplasia.
- **Surgical excision** allows for pathologic evaluation of histology and invasion. May have high morbidity from vaginal stenosis or shortening.

The appearance of sarcoma botryoides is commonly described as a "bunch of grapes" protruding from introitus of a young child or infant.

TABLE 6-8. Treatment Options for Squamous Cell Vaginal Cancer by Stage

STAGE	TREATMENT
I	Intracavitary or interstitial radiation therapy or radical vaginectomy
IIA	Whole pelvic irradiation with intracavitary irradiation or radical surgery
IIB, III, IV	Whole pelvic irradiation with parametrial boost
Recurrent	Anterior, posterior, or total exenteration

- **Ablation** with CO_2 laser may be used for low or moderate dysplasia. Generally well tolerated. May require multiple treatments.
- **Intracavitary radiation** reserved for patients who have failed or are not candidates for other treatment or who have extensive, multifocal disease.

VAGINAL CARCINOMA

Squamous cell therapy determined by stage, location, and patient preference:

- See Table 6–8 for a list of treatment options based on stage.
- Radiation is mainstay of treatment.
- Surgery not commonly chosen because the degree of resection necessary for negative margins often results in a nonfunctional vagina.
- Surgery may provide good results for patients with small, stage I disease and may be necessary in cases where fistulas have developed.
- 5 year survival rates are found in Table 6–9.

Verrucous carcinoma is treated by surgical resection as it is not responsive to radiation or chemotherapy. Often recurs following surgery, but rarely metastatic.

Malignant melanoma has an extremely poor prognosis. Treatment is surgical resection.

Clear cell adenocarcinoma is treated with intracavitary or transvaginal irradiation. Often requires radical hysterectomy, vaginectomy, and lymphadenectomy. 5-year survival is 90% for stage I and 80% for stage II lesions.

TABLE 6-9. Survival Rates for Squamous Cell Carcinoma of the Vagina

STAGE	1-YEAR SURVIVAL	2-YEAR SURVIVAL	5-YEAR SURVIVAL
I	91%	88%	73%
II	78%	64%	51%
III	63%	40%	33%
IVA	48%	30%	20%
IVB	33%	0%	0%

- Least common site of gynecologic malignancy
- BRCA 1 or BRCA 2 mutation carriers have a 120-fold increased risk, which is decreased substantially with prophylactic bilateral salpingo-oophorectomy.
- Spread by transcoelomic exfoliation of cells that implant throughout peritoneal cavity and lymphatic drainage.
- CA125 serves as a tumor marker.

DIAGNOSIS

Classic triad is colicky pain, abnormal bleeding, and leukorrhea (seen in 15%). Abnormal bleeding is most common symptom. Criteria for diagnosis includes:

- Main tumor in tube, arising from endosalpinx
- Histology pattern usually papillary, reproduces epithelium
- If wall involved, benign, and malignant transition should be identifiable
- Ovaries and endometrium normal or less tumor involvement than tube

Histology

Histology similar to papillary serous carcinoma of ovary in 90% of cases, but can be endometrioid, clear cell, adenosquamous, squamous cell, sarcoma, choriocarcinoma, malignant teratoma.

Staging

Staging is surgical. See Table 6–18 for staging criteria.

TREATMENT AND SURVIVAL

- Treatment is surgical cytoreduction and chemotherapy (carboplatin and paclitaxel).
- Residual disease after cytoreduction is a good predictor of survival rate.
- 5-year survival rates are:
  - Overall: 56%
  - Stage I: 84%
  - Stage II: 52%
  - Stage III: 36%

Gestational trophoblastic disease (GTD) can be **benign** (hydatidaform molar pregnancy) or **malignant** (invasive trophoblastic disease, choriocarcinoma, placental site trophoblastic tumors).

RISK FACTORS FOR GTD INCLUDE:

- Age <20 or >35
- Lack of prior delivery
- Prior spontaneous abortion

- History of prior molar pregnancy
- Dietary factors (vitamin A deficiency or low carotene)

Benign GTD

HYDATIDIFORM MOLAR PREGNANCY

- Complete hydatidiform mole (complete HM) and partial hydatidaform mole (partial HM) are types of benign GTD.
- Complete HM are "completely" composed of paternal chromosomes. See Table 6–10 for a comparison of findings.
- **Incidence** is 1 in 1000. In women >50 years it occurs in 1 out of 3 pregnancies.

Complete HM are "completely dad's fault"–they contain only paternal chromosomes.

SYMPTOMS

Partial HM often asymptomatic and presents as missed or incomplete abortion. Symptoms more common in complete HM pregnancy and include:
- Vaginal bleeding
- Uterine size greater than dates
- Preeclampsia <20 weeks gestation
- Theca lutein cysts (more likely if markedly elevated hCG)
- Hyperemesis gravidarum (more likely if markedly elevated hCG)

TABLE 6–10. Pathologic Characteristics of Hydatidiform Molar Pregnancies

	PATHOLOGIC FINDINGS	CLINICAL FINDINGS
Complete HM	■ Large, diffusely hydropic villi ■ Absence of fetal tissue ■ Cisterns often present ■ Scalloped villi with stromal trophoblastic inclusions are rare ■ 46XX (90%). Fertilization of empty or inactivated egg by haploid sperm that duplicates ■ 46XY (10%). Fertilization of egg by two sperm	■ 5–20% associated with invasive disease or **choriocarcinoma** ■ Associated with medical complications ■ Serum hCG >100,000
Partial HM	■ Large hydropic villi mixed with normal or small for gestational age villi ■ Presence of fetal tissue ■ Cisterns may be present, but less prominent ■ Scalloped villi with stromal trophoblastic inclusions ■ 69XXY or 69XYY (90%). Fertilization of haploid ovum by two haploid sperm	■ 4% associated with invasive disease ■ Rarely associated with medical complications ■ Serum hCG <100,000

- Hyperthyroidism (more likely if markedly elevated hCG)
- Passage of hydropic vesicles from vagina

DIAGNOSIS

- Quantitative serum β-hCG elevated above expected for gestational age
- Ultrasound findings:
    - Complete HM—no fetal tissue or amniotic fluid, "**snowstorm pattern**" seen
    - Partial HM—fetal tissue present, focal cystic spaces in placenta. Increased echogenicity of villi, increased transverse diameter of gestational sac
- Preoperative studies: Pelvic ultrasound, urinalysis, CXR, labs (CBC, hCG, coagulation studies, chemistry panel, thyroid function tests)

Complete HM are more likely to be symptomatic. Partial HM usually presents as a missed or incomplete spontaneous abortion.

TREATMENT

- Treatment is usually evacuation of the uterus by suction curettage.
- Hysterectomy offered if future fertility not desired.
- Prophylactic chemotherapy (methotrexate or actinomycin D) considered in high risk complete HM or in patients unlikely to comply with follow-up.
- See Table 6–11 for a list of risk factors.

FOLLOW-UP

- Serum hCG every 2 weeks until three consecutive negative levels, then monthly serum hCG for 6–12 months.
- Avoidance of pregnancy for 6 months after the first normal hCG.
- Placenta from all future pregnancies should be sent for pathologic evaluation.
- hCG levels 6 weeks after completion of all future pregnancies.
- History of complete or partial HM does not increase risk for antepartum or intrapartum complications with future pregnancies.

Malignant GTD

Malignant GTD usually occurs after a molar pregnancy, but can also occur after a spontaneous or induced abortion, ectopic pregnancy, or normal intrauterine pregnancy.

INVASIVE GESTATIONAL TROPHOBLASTIC DISEASE

Occurs in 20% of patients with complete HM and 4% of patients with partial HM. Lesions spread through direct extension and may metastasize through vascular channels.

TABLE 6-11. **Risk Factors for Invasive Gestational Trophoblastic Disease**

- Uterine size >20 weeks
- Age >40 years
- Theca lutein cysts >6 cm
- hCG >100,000 IU/L
- Prior HM
- Medical complications from molar pregnancy
- Poor involution of uterus with hemorrhage after evacuation

SYMPTOMS

- Often no symptoms
- Vaginal bleeding (common)
- Symptoms secondary to metastatic disease (hemoptysis, abdominal pain, hematochezia, melena, neurological defects)

DIAGNOSIS

- Plateau or rise in hCG levels after molar pregnancy, failure of hCG to normalize 6 months after evacuation, or hCG >20,000 mIU/mL 4 weeks after evacuation
- Repeat uterine curettage with molar tissue
- Molar tissue at metastatic sites (15% are metastatic, usually to lung and vagina)
- Workup: hCG, CBC, chemistry panel, liver function tests, coagulation studies, thyroid function tests, pelvic ultrasound, CT or MRI of abdomen and pelvis, CT or x-ray of chest, CT or MRI of brain if has vaginal or lung metastasis

TREATMENT

- Hysterectomy for nonmetastatic disease
- Single agent chemotherapy (methotrexate or actinomycin D) if low risk or desires future fertility
- Multiagent chemotherapy if high risk or refractory to single agent. Regimen is EMA/CO (Etoposide, Methotrexate, Actinomycin D, Leukovorin, Cyclophosphamide, Vincristine)

Choriocarcinoma

Extremely malignant tumor arising from any source of trophoblastic tissue:

- 50% after molar pregnancy
- 25% after abortion or ectopic pregnancy
- 25% after normal term pregnancy

SYMPTOMS

- Irregular or late postpartum bleeding
- Enlarged uterus
- Ovarian masses
- Symptoms secondary to metastatic disease (lung, brain, liver)

DIAGNOSIS

- Same workup as for invasive gestational trophoblastic disease.
- Incidence of metastases at diagnosis is 15–25%.

TREATMENT

- Single-agent chemotherapy (Methotrexate or Actinomycin D) if low–risk patients.
- Multiagent chemotherapy (EMA/CO) for high-risk patients (WHO score ≥7). See Table IV for WHO scoring system.

Placental Site Trophoblastic Tumor

- Extremely rare tumor composed of intermediate cytotrophoblastic cells.
- Usually occurs after normal term pregnancy.
- Tends to stay confined to uterus, with metastasis only late in disease.

SYMPTOMS

- Irregular vaginal bleeding (menorrhagia, metrorrhagia, or amenorrhea)
- Enlarged uterus
- Virilization (from ovarian hyperthecosis)
- Nephrotic syndrome

DIAGNOSIS

- Workup as for invasive GTD (see Gestational Trophoblastic Disease section).
- Serum hCG may be normal or only minimally elevated.

TREATMENT

- Hysterectomy is first-line treatment because not very responsive to chemotherapy.
- Chemotherapy with EMA/CO or EMA/EP.

COMPARISON OF MALIGNANT GTDs

Pathologic characteristics of malignant GTDs are outlined in Table 6–12.

FOLLOW-UP OF MALIGNANT GTD

After chemotherapy, follow-up for malignant GTD is:

- Serum hCG every 1–2 weeks for 3 months
- Serum hCG monthly for 12 months
- Avoidance of pregnancy for 12 months after completion of treatment
- Placenta from all future pregnancies should be sent for pathologic evaluation
- hCG levels 6 weeks after completion of all future pregnancies

TABLE 6–12. **Pathologic Characteristics of Gestational Trophoblastic Neoplasias**

	PATHOLOGIC FINDINGS
Invasive GTD	- Enlarged villi - Invasion into myometrium - Presence of molar tissue found at metastatic sites
Choriocarcinoma	- Absent villi - Extensive myometrial invasion and destruction - Malignant cytotrophoblasts and syncytiotrophoblasts - Cut surface red/brown and beefy with extensive hemorrhage and necrosis
Placental site trophoblastic tumor	- Intermediate trophoblastic cells - Cells infiltrating myometrium at site of placental implantation - Cut surface tan, yellow or white. May have focal or extensive hemorrhage

TABLE 6–13. World Health Organization (WHO) Scoring System

RISK FACTOR	SCORE			
	0	1	2	4
Age (years)	</= 39	>40		
Antecedent pregnancy	Hydatidiform mole	Abortion	Term	
Interval of pregnancy to start of treatment (months)	<4	4–6	7–12	>12
hCG (mIU/mL)	<1000	1000–10,000	10,000–100,000	>100,000
Largest tumor mass (cm)	<3	3–5	>5	
Site of metastasis	None or other sites	Spleen, kidney	Gastrointestinal tract	Brain, liver
Number of metastasis	0	1–4	5–8	>8
Prior chemotherapy			Single drug	≥2 drugs

PROGNOSIS OF GTD

Prognosis is dependent on risk factors. Risk factors and the WHO scoring system is found in Table 6–13. Total score ≤4 is low risk, 5–7 intermediate risk, and ≥8 high risk.

▶ PAIN MANAGEMENT

- Majority of patients (90%) with terminal cancer can have satisfactory relief.
- Most important goal is optimization of quality of life.
- Many patients are depressed, which exacerbates perception of pain.
- Multistep approach (overlap of medications to minimize side effects):
  - Anti-inflammatory medications
  - Opioids
  - Antidepressants
  - Corticosteroids
  - Neuroleptics (carbamazepine, valproic acid)

▶ PALLIATIVE CARE

Palliative care requires multispecialty coordination. It is important to reassure patients that it does not mean abandonment. Three main intents are:

- Minimizing pain
- Optimization of quality of life
- Forgoing life-sustaining intervention

186

Modalities of Palliative Care

- **Medical management** used to treat common symptoms of nausea, vomiting, constipation, weight loss, pain, depression.
- **Radiation** therapy used to control severe vaginal bleeding from primary or metastatic malignancies to prevent pain and suffering from exsanguination.
- **Surgical therapy** may be necessary for relief from bowel obstruction. The patient must be aware of the risks, benefits, and impact on quality of life.

Do Not Resuscitate Indications and Implications

- Do not resuscitate (DNR) orders indicated when it is likely that patient is near the end of life.
- Process should involve family, physicians, often clergy.
- Most important principles: **Informed consent** and **autonomy.**

► **SEXUAL ISSUES**

- Gynecologic and breast cancer affect a woman's sexuality and well-being.
- Spread of disease, surgical, and radiation treatment can result in infertility, stomas, disfigurement, alopecia, inability to have intercourse.
- Patients should be approached and offered medical treatment, support groups, counselors.

► **CANCER STAGING**

VULVAR CARCINOMA

Vulvar carcinoma is **surgically staged.** See Table 6–14 for staging definitions.

VAGINAL CARCINOMA

Vaginal carcinoma is **clinically staged.** See Table 6–15 for staging definitions.

CERVICAL CARCINOMA

Cervical carcinoma is **clinically staged.** See Table 6–16 for staging definitions.

UTERINE CARCINOMA

- Uterine carcinoma is **surgically staged.**
- Grade or histology differentiation always included in staging. Grade classification:
  - Grade 1: ≤5% of a nonsquamous/nonmorular solid growth pattern
  - Grade 2: 6–50% of a nonsquamous/nonmorular solid growth pattern
  - Grade 3: >50% of a nonsquamous/nonmolecular social growth pattern

See Table 6–17 for staging definitions.

TABLE 6–14. Vulvar Carcinoma Staging System

STAGE	DEFINITION
I	Confined to vulva or perineum, ≤**2 cm**
IA	Stromal invasion ≤1 cm
IB	Stromal invasion >1 mm
II	Confined to vulva or perineum, >**2 cm**
III	Tumor any size with extension to: —Adjacent spread to lower urethra, vagina, or anus —Unilateral regional lymph node metastasis
IV	Extension or pelvic lymph node metastasis
IVA	Invasion to upper urethra, bladder mucosa, rectal mucosa, pelvic bone, or bilateral regional nodes
IVB	Distant metastases or pelvic lymph nodes

FALLOPIAN TUBE CARCINOMA

Fallopian tube carcinoma is **surgically staged.** See Table 6–18 for staging definitions.

OVARIAN CARCINOMA

Ovarian carcinoma is **surgically staged.** See Table 6–19 for staging definitions.

GESTATIONAL TROPHOBLASTIC CARCINOMA

Gestational trophoblastic carcinoma is **surgically staged.** See Table 6–20 for staging definitions.

TABLE 6–15. Vaginal Carcinoma Staging System

STAGE	DEFINITION
I	Limited to vaginal wall
II	Involves subvaginal tissue, no extension to pelvic wall
III	Extension to pelvic wall
IV	Extension beyond true pelvis, bladder invasion, rectum invasion
IVA	Bladder or rectal mucosa invasion Direct extension beyond true pelvis
IVB	Distant metastases

TABLE 6–16. Cervical Cancer Staging System

STAGE	DEFINITION
I	**Confined to cervix only**
IA	Microscopic lesion, extension ≤7 mm
IA1	Stromal invasion depth ≤3mm
IA2	Stromal invasion depth between 3–5 mm
IB	Microscopic larger than IA or any macroscopic (clinically visible)
IB1	Microscopic with extension >7 mm or depth >5 mm or macroscopic but ≤4 cm
IB2	Macroscopic >4 cm
II	**Extends beyond cervix, but not to pelvic sidewall or lower 2/3 of vagina**
IIA	Extends to upper 2/3 of vagina, no parametrial involvement
IIB	Parametrial involvement
III	**Extends to lower 1/3 of vagina or pelvic side wall**
IIIA	Extends to lower 1/3 of vagina, but not to pelvic side wall
IIIB	Extends to pelvic side wall or evidence of hydronephrosis or nonfunctioning kidney
IV	**Extends beyond true pelvis, involves bladder, or rectal mucosa**
IVA	Spread to adjacent organs (bladder or rectum)
IVB	Distant metastases

TABLE 6–17. Uterine Cancer Staging System

STAGE	DEFINITION
I	**Uterine corpus only**
IA	Limited to endometrium
IB	Invasion <50% of myometrium
IC	Invasion ≥50% of myometrium
II	**Involvement of cervix**
IIA	Endocervical glandular involvement only

TABLE 6–17.   Uterine Cancer Staging System (*Continued*)

STAGE	DEFINITION
IIB	Cervical stromal invasion
III	**Invasion beyond the cervix/corpus**
IIIA	Invades uterine serosa and/or adnexa, and/or positive peritoneal washings
IIIB	Metastases to the vagina
IIIC	Metastases to the pelvic or para-aortic lymph nodes
IV	**Distant metastases or metastases to adjacent organs**
IVA	Bladder/bowel mucosa invasion
IVB	Distant metastases including intraabdominal and/or inguinal lymph nodes

TABLE 6–18.   Fallopian Tube Cancer Staging System

STAGE	DEFINITION
0	**Carcinoma in situ** (limited to tubal mucosa)
I	**Limited to fallopian tubes**
IA	Involves one fallopian tube only, not penetrating serosal surface
IB	Involves both fallopian tubes, not penetrating serosal surface
IC	Tumor extends through or onto tubal serosa or positive peritoneal washings or ascites
II	**Extension into the pelvis**
IIA	Extension or metastases to uterus or ovaries
IIB	Extension to other pelvic tissues
IIC	IIA or IIB with tumor on tubal serosa or positive peritoneal washings or ascites
III	**Peritoneal implants outside pelvis (including superficial liver mets), abdominal nodal involvement, or invasion into bowel**
IIIA	Microscopic histologically confirmed peritoneal spread, but no gross tumor outside of the pelvis and negative nodes
IIIB	Macroscopic (gross) histologically confirmed peritoneal spread ≤ 2 cm; lymph nodes negative
IIIC	Peritoneal implants >2 cm or positive pelvic, para-aortic, inguinal lymph nodes
IV	**Distant metastases,** or parenchymal liver metastases, or pleural effusion with positive cytology

TABLE 6–19. Ovarian Cancer Staging System

STAGE	DEFINITION
I	**Limited to ovaries**
IA	Involves one ovary only, capsule intact
IB	Involves both ovaries, capsules intact
IC	Tumor present on surface of ovary, capsule ruptured, or positive peritoneal washings
II	**Extension into the pelvis**
IIA	Extension or metastases to uterus or fallopian tubes
IIB	Extension to other pelvic tissues
IIC	IIA or IIB with tumor on surface of ovary, capsule ruptured, or positive peritoneal washings
III	**Peritoneal implants outside pelvis (including superficial liver mets), abdominal nodal involvement, or invasion into bowel**
IIIA	Microscopic histologically confirmed peritoneal spread, but no gross tumor outside of the pelvis and negative nodes
IIIB	Macroscopic (gross) histologically confirmed peritoneal spread ≤2 cm; lymph nodes negative
IIIC	Peritoneal implants >2 cm or positive pelvic, para-aortic, inguinal lymph nodes
IV	**Distant metastases**

TABLE 6–20. Gestational Trophoblastic Disease Staging System

STAGE	DEFINITION
I	Confined to uterus
II	Extension outside of uterus, but limited to genital structures
III	Extends to lungs, with or without genital tract involvement
IV	All other metastatic sites (brain, liver)

CHAPTER 7

Primary and Preventive Care

Jeannine Rahimian, MD, MBA
Julie Henriksen, MD, FACOG

Basic Ethical Concepts

- **Autonomy:** Respect for the patient's right to make their own choices.
- **Beneficence:** Duty to promote the good of the patient. The welfare of the patient is central to all considerations.
- **Justice:** Avoidance of discrimination on the basis of race, color, religion, national origin, or any basis that would be discriminatory.
- **Nonmalfeasance:** The duty not to inflict harm or injury (do no harm).
- **Paternalism:** Imposing a mandate or interfering for perceived good of patient.
- **Positive rights:** Right to be provided with something through another person or state (i.e., right to education or health care).
- **Negative rights:** Right not to be subjected to an action usually in the form of coercion (i.e., freedom of speech or freedom from violent crime).

Informed Consent

- Process by which fully informed patient participates in making health-care choices.
- Patient should understand:
    - Diagnosis
    - Recommended treatment
    - Potential complications (risks and benefits)
    - Alternative options
- Should assess patient's understanding and acceptance of intervention or treatment.

Advanced Directive

- Written description of a patient's choice for treatment in the event they are unable to communicate their wishes directly.
- Types of advanced directives include:
    - **Living will**—takes effect when terminally ill.
    - **Durable power of attorney**—identifies an individual who has authority to make health-care decisions if they are unable to do so.
    - **Do not resuscitate order (DNR)**—request not to have cardiopulmonary resuscitation (CPR) or intubation in event of cardiac or respiratory failure.

- Sets security standards for protecting the confidentiality and privacy of patients' health information.
- Limits sharing of health information to those involved with an individual patient's care, the patient, and family members if specified.
- Limits release of mental health records.

Definitions

- Precision is the ability of a measurement to be constantly reproduced. Precision does not imply accuracy.

PRIMARY AND PREVENTIVE CARE

- Accuracy is the degree to which a measurement represents the true value of that which is being measured.
- Incidence is the number of instances an illness is identified within a given period of time.
- Prevalence is the number of instances of an illness in a given population at a designated time.
- Relative risk is the ratio of risk of disease in those exposed to the risk of disease in those not exposed (RR >1.0 signifies a positive association between exposure and disease).
- Odds ratio is a way of comparing whether the probability of a certain exposure having occurred is the same for two groups. It is the ratio of the odds in favor of exposure among those with disease (a/b) to odds in favor of exposure in those without disease (c/d). It can also be calculated as ad/bc on Table 7–1.
- Evidence-based medicine is the conscientious and judicious use of current best evidence in health-care decision making.

Types of Studies

RANDOMIZED CLINICAL TRIAL

- Participants randomly assigned to exposure or nonexposure groups
- Intervention applied and outcomes measured (preferably blinded)
- Advantages:
  - Able to avoid selection bias and confounding
  - Greatest ability to assess causality
- Disadvantages:
  - Expense, feasibility
  - Ethical issues of assigning placebo for certain problems

COHORT STUDY

- Observational study of large numbers over a long period of time
- Comparison of incidence rates in groups that differ in exposure levels
- Usually prospective
- Disadvantages:
  - More subject to systematic error
  - Since not randomized, likelihood that two groups are equal at baseline is lower

CASE CONTROL STUDY

- Observational study of patients with disease compared to those without disease to determine association between exposure and disease.

TABLE 7–1. Calculation of Odds Ratio

	EXPOSED (+)	NOT EXPOSED (−)
Disease (+)	a	b
No disease (−)	c	d

- Retrospective study.
- Advantages:
    - Highly efficient, often requiring fewest number of patients to demonstrate an association
    - Requires less time and money than other studies
- Disadvantages:
    - Retrospective
    - Relies on patient recall (recall bias)
    - Knowledge of health outcome may influence interpretation of data (observer bias)

CROSS-SECTIONAL STUDY

- Observational study of individuals with and without disease and examines relationship to variables.
- "Snapshot" of group of individuals at any given time and analysis of disease and variable of interest.

META-ANALYSIS

- Combining data of multiple trials
- Aggregation of data

DECISION ANALYSIS

- Quantitative approach to evaluate relative value of management options.
- Clinical problem is broken down into options, and tree or algorithm created.
- Probability values for each parameter are estimated from literature and net value for each decision is calculated.

ECONOMIC ANALYSIS

- Systematic review similar to decision analysis, but focuses on monetary cost.
- Compares costs of different options to determine best care for least cost.
- Difficult to put monetary value of clinical outcome.

Sensitivity and Specificity

- Sensitivity is:
    - Proportion of people who have disease who are identified as having disease by the screening test.
    - Calculated as $a/(a + c)$ on Table 7–2.
- Specificity is:
    - Proportion of people without disease who are identified as not having disease by the screening test.
    - Calculated as $d/(b + d)$ on Table 7–2.
- Sensitivity and specificity is a function of the screening test and is independent of prevalence of disease in population being tested.

Predictive Value

- Positive predictive value is:
    - Probability that person with positive test result has the disease.
    - Calculated as $a/(a + b)$ on Table 7–2.

TABLE 7-2. Sensitivity and Specificity Analysis: True Status

	DISEASE (+)	NO DISEASE (−)	TOTAL
Test positive (+)	a	b	a + b
Test negative (−)	c	d	c + d
Total	a + c	b + d	a + b + c + d

a = individuals with disease who test positive (true positive)
b = individuals without disease who test positive (false positive)
c = individuals with disease who test negative (false negative)
d = individuals without disease who test negative (true negative)

- Negative predictive value is:
  - Probability that person with negative test result does not have the disease.
  - Calculated as $d/(c + d)$ on Table 7–2.
- Positive and negative predictive value will change based on prevalence of the disease in the population being tested.

Errors in Epidemiology

- Type I error (α) is when a statistically significant difference is found when there is no actual difference:
  - Based on choice of level of statistical significance (P value)
  - A P value of <0.05 defines that the possibility that the finding was due to chance is 5%
- Type II error (β) is when no statistically significant difference is found when a difference actually does exist
  - The "power" of a study is its ability to detect an association
  - The larger the power of a study, the smaller the chance of a type II error.

▶ PRACTICE MANAGEMENT

Health-Care Financing Methods

- Self-payment:
  - Patient pays "out-of-pocket" full fees as set by physician or practice.
- Preferred provider organization (PPO):
  - More flexible than health maintenance organization (HMO), as allows patient to see specialist without referral by primary-care physician (PCP).
  - Out-of-network physician coverage is usually less, such that the patient has an incentive to stay within network.
- Health maintenance organization (HMO):
  - Patients identify PCP and are required to use participating or approved providers.
  - Require referral from PCP to be seen by a specialist.
- Prepaid health-care plan:
  - Voluntary health plan where the patient can prepay monthly fees that will go to cover medical expenses as they arise.
  - Rising health-care costs have made this type of coverage inadequate.

- Private health insurance:
  - Insurance purchased by an individual or family
  - Allows patient to be seen at any hospital or by any provider
  - Usually more expensive
- Managed care organization (MCO)
  - Group of providers who receive capitated (per member per month) payment and agree to deliver health-care services as defined by the contract.
  - Term often used to refer to all forms of health-care organizations (PPO, HMO, POS).

Health-Care Management Terms

- Utilization:
  - Amount of used services of hospital care, physician services, and prescription coverage
  - Usually referred to as dollars of expenditure
- Capitation:
  - Specified monthly payment given to provider to provide defined services.
  - Payments usually made as per member per month and fixed regardless of actual cost required to provide health-care services.
- Risk sharing:
  - Distribution of financial risk among various parties involved in providing health care.
  - Example would be hospital and physician group agreeing to share financial risk if expenses exceed revenue.

▶ RISK MANAGEMENT

Malpractice Insurance

- Types of professional liability:
  - Occurrence policy: Covers losses that occur during period of coverage no matter when the loss is reported.
  - Claims made policy: Covers claims made during period of coverage no matter when the loss occurred. Usually less expensive than occurrence policy.
  - Tail coverage: Purchased after claims made policy terminated to cover claims that may arise from previous losses. Claims made and tail coverage together act like an occurrence policy.

Malpractice Claims

- Most common reasons for malpractice claims:
  - Inadequate rapport or communication
  - Failure or delay in diagnosing a specific disorder
  - Failure to obtain timely consultation
  - Failure to obtain informed consent
  - Negligent performance of a procedure
  - Negligent treatment with medication
  - Poor documentation of medical care

Medico-Legal Terms

- Standard of care:
  - Level at which an average, prudent health-care provider would manage a given patient or health-care issue.

- Breach of standard of care:
  - Health-care provider not providing health-care management or treatment at the level at which an average, prudent health-care provider would.
- Proximate cause of injury:
  - An event sufficiently related to a legally recognizable injury that it can be considered to be the cause of the injury.
- Intentional tort:
  - Intentional act that is reasonably foreseeable to cause harm to an individual and that does so.
- Negligent tort
  - Provider breaches a prudent duty of care that was the proximate cause of injury and resulted in damages to the patient.

▶ PERIODIC HEALTH ASSESSMENT

Leading Causes of Death by Age

- Age 13–18:
  1. Motor vehicle accidents
  2. Homicide
  3. Suicide
  4. Cancer
- Age 19–39:
  1. Accidents and adverse effects
  2. Human immunodeficiency virus
  3. Cancer
  4. Diseases of the heart
- Age 40–64:
  1. Cancer
  2. Diseases of the heart
  3. Cerebrovascular diseases
  4. Accidents and adverse effects
- Age 65 and older:
  1. Diseases of the heart
  2. Cancer
  3. Cerebrovascular diseases
  4. Chronic obstructive pulmonary diseases

Routine and High-Risk Screening

CHOLESTEROL TESTING

- Routine: Lipid testing every 5 years beginning at age 45
- Earlier screening if high risk, defined as:
  - Coronary heart disease
  - Diabetes mellitus (DM)
  - Familial lipid disorders
  - Family history of premature coronary heart disease

COLORECTAL CANCER SCREENING

- Routine screening starting at age 50 with:
  - Sigmoidoscopy every 5 years with annual fecal occult blood testing **or**

- Colonoscopy every 10 years **or**
- Double contrast barium enema every 5–10 years
- Earlier initiation if high risk, defined as:
  - History of adenomatous polyps or inflammatory bowel disease
  - Colorectal cancer in first-degree relative <60 years
  - Family history of familial adenomatous polyposis or nonpolyposis colon cancer

FASTING GLUCOSE TESTING

- Routine: Every 3 years after age 45
- Earlier and more frequent screening if high risk, defined as:
  - Obesity
  - First-degree relative with diabetes
  - History of gestational diabetes
  - Hypertension
  - High-risk ethnic population (African American, Hispanic, Asian, Pacific Islander, Native American)

HEMOGLOBIN LEVEL

- Testing only recommended in high risk, defined as:
  - History of excessive menstrual flow
  - Caribbean, Latin American, Asian, Mediterranean, or African ancestry

HUMAN IMMUNODEFICIENCY VIRUS (HIV) TESTING

- Testing should be done in high-risk individuals, defined as:
  - Seeking treatment for sexually transmitted disease
  - Intravenous (IV) drug user
  - Multiple sexual partners
  - Men who have sex with men
  - Past or present partner with HIV or IV drug use
  - History of blood transfusion between 1978 and 1985
  - Invasive cervical cancer
  - All pregnant women
  - Patients in a population where the HIV prevalence is ≥1%
  - Patients in institutionalized settings such as correctional facilities, homeless shelters
  - Patients in TB clinics

MAMMOGRAPHY

- Routine screening with mammography:
  - Every 1–2 years starting at age 40
  - Annually after age 50
- Earlier screening recommended in high risk, defined as:
  - First-degree relative (mother, sister, daughter) with breast cancer
  - Multiple relatives with premenopausal breast or ovarian cancer

THYROID STIMULATING HORMONE (TSH) TESTING

- Screening of high risk patients, defined as:
  - Strong family history of thyroid disease
  - Autoimmune disease

TUBERCULOSIS SKIN TESTING

- Should test high-risk patients, defined as:
  - HIV positive
  - Close contact with person with tuberculosis
  - Low income, medically underserved
  - Alcoholism or IV drug use
  - Resident of long-term facility
  - Health-care professionals working in high-risk facilities

Immunizations

HEPATITIS A VACCINATION

- High-risk groups should be offered vaccination. They include:
  - International travelers
  - Illegal drug users
  - Chronic liver disease patients
  - Clotting factor disorders
  - Sex partners of men who have sex with men
  - Food service, day-care or health-care workers

HEPATITIS B VACCINATION

- Should be offered to:
  - International travelers
  - IV drug users and their sexual contacts
  - Chronic renal or liver disease patients
  - Clotting factor disorders
  - Sex partners of men who have sex with men
  - Health-care workers
  - Household or sexual contact with hepatitis B carrier

INFLUENZA VACCINATION

- Should be offered to:
  - Resident of long-term care facility
  - Chronic cardiopulmonary disorders
  - Health-care or day-care workers
  - Pregnant women who will be in second or third trimester during epidemic season
  - Ages 50 and above
  - Metabolic disorders (DM, hemoglobinopathies, immunosuppression, renal dysfunction)

MEASLES MUMPS RUBELLA VACCINATION

- Should be offered to:
  - Adults born in or after 1957
  - Health-care workers
  - Students entering college
  - International travelers
  - Rubella negative postpartum patients
  - Immunocompromised

PNEUMOCOCCAL VACCINATION

- Should be offered to patients with:
    - Chronic illness such as asthma, cardiovascular disease, DM, alcoholism, chronic liver disease
    - Immunocompromised (HIV, malignancies, chemotherapy, steroid therapy)
    - Pregnant patients with chronic illness
    - Asplenia
    - Recent pneumonia

TETANUS VACCINATION

- TdaP (tetanus, diphtheria, acellular pertussis) as booster every 10 years and for caregivers of infants

▶ OTITIS MEDIA

SIGNS AND SYMPTOMS

- Ear pain
- Ear fullness
- Decreased hearing

DIAGNOSIS

- Erythematous, bulging tympanic membrane

TREATMENT

- Amoxicillin for 10–14 days
- For penicillin allergic, should give trimethoprim-sulfamethoxazole (TMP-SMX) or macrolides

▶ ALLERGIC RHINITIS

- May be seasonal or perennial
- Incidence greatest in adolescence

SIGNS AND SYMPTOMS

- Sneezing, nasal itching, nasal congestion
- Sore throat, throat clearing, itching of throat and palate
- Conjunctivitis with ocular itching, lacrimation, and puffiness
- Sleep disturbance, association with obstructive sleep apnea

DIAGNOSIS

- Swollen nasal turbinates with pale or bluish mucosa
- Clear nasal discharge and secretions along posterior wall of oropharynx
- Conjuctival erythema
- Dark circles under eyes

DIFFERENTIAL DIAGNOSIS

- Nonallergic rhinitis (infectious, vasomotor)
- Overuse of nasal sprays
- Hormonal (i.e., pregnancy related or with OCP use)
- Drug induced (cocaine, α- and β-blockers)
- Structural abnormality

TREATMENT

- Avoidance of allergens or allergen immunotherapy
- Antihistamines—most effective if used regularly
- Oral decongestants
- Intranasal steroids—most effective when used regularly

▶ RESPIRATORY TRACT INFECTIONS

Upper Respiratory Tract Infection

Viral or bacterial infection of the nares, sinuses, pharynx, or inner ear

SYMPTOMS

- Runny nose, congestion, sinus pain, scratchy sore throat, ear pain, mild fever

DIFFERENTIAL DIAGNOSIS

- Bacterial sinusitis
- Bacterial pharyngitis
- Mononucleosis
- Otitis media

DIAGNOSIS

- Routine imaging not necessary for uncomplicated upper respiratory tract infection (URI), otitis media, or sinusitis
- Pharnygeal swab for group A streptococci if indicated

TREATMENT

- Treat symptoms—rest, fluids, nonsteroidal anti-inflammatory (NSAIDs), salt-water gargle, over-the-counter decongestants

Bronchitis

SIGNS AND SYMPTOMS

- Productive or nonproductive cough for 1–3 weeks.
- Lung examination may be normal or include wheezes and rhonchi.
- Typically no egophony or dullness to percussion.

DIFFERENTIAL DIAGNOSIS

- Community-acquired pneumonia
- Reactive airway disease (asthma)

DIAGNOSIS

- Diagnosis based on history and examination.
- Chest x-ray (CXR) **not routinely indicated** except in patient with chronic or nonresolving symptoms.

TREATMENT

- Antibiotics not indicated since viral etiology
- Expectorants and over-the-counter decongestants
- Bronchodilators (albuterol inhaler)

Pneumonia

SIGNS AND SYMPTOMS

- Productive cough, fever, shortness of breath, chest tightness, or pain
- Mild or no distress
- Wheezes or rhonchi
- Focal decreased breath sounds, egophony, dullness to percussion

DIFFERENTIAL DIAGNOSIS

- Viral bronchitis
- Influenza
- URI

DIAGNOSIS

- Clinical history and examination should suggest need for CXR
- Pulse oximetry to measure oxygen saturation
- Consider blood cultures if febrile

TREATMENT

- Macrolides or fluoroquinolones

Tuberculosis

SYMPTOMS

- Fever, cough, chills, respiratory distress
- Pleuritic chest pain
- Weight loss
- Night sweats

DIAGNOSIS

- Focal findings, clinical suspicion or positive PPD warrant CXR.
- All pregnant patients and patients at risk of TB should be screened.

TABLE 7–3.   **Treatment of TB**

TB Prophylaxis—new PPD+, negative CXR	Isoniazid 300 mg/day for 6–12 months
	or
	Rifampin 600 mg/day for 4 months if INH-resistant strain suspected
	6 months treatment with one of the following regimens:
Active TB or	Isoniazid + Rifampin + Pyrazinamide **or**
Reactivation TB or	Isoniazid +Rifampin + Pyrazinamide + Ethambutol **or**
Miliary TB (extra-pulmonary TB)	Isoniazid + Rifampin + Pyrazinamide + Streptomycin

TREATMENT (HIV-NEGATIVE PATIENTS)

■ Treatment depends on stage of tuberculosis identified. See Table 7–3.

▶ ASTHMA

■ Chronic inflammatory disorder resulting in airway hyperresponsiveness

SIGNS AND SYMPTOMS

■ Dyspnea at rest or with exertion
■ Cough
■ Wheezing
■ Chest tightness
■ Awakening at night with symptoms

DIAGNOSIS

■ Expiratory wheezing, prolonged expiratory phase, increased respiratory rate.
■ Signs of allergic rhinitis such as boggy nasal mucosa, cobblestoning of posterior oropharynx, swelling under eyes.
■ Pulmonary function tests:
    ■ Decreased FEV_1/FVC ratio
    ■ Reversible obstruction—increase in FEV_1 after bronchodilator
    ■ Normal diffusion capacity

TREATMENT

ACUTE ASTHMA

■ Inhaled β-agonists
■ Monitoring of oxygen saturation and peak flow
■ If incomplete response with β-agonists, treatment with systemic corticosteroids

CHRONIC ASTHMA

■ Short acting inhaled β-agonists as needed.
■ If requires bronchodilator use ≥2 times per week, may need other therapy such as:

- Low dose inhaled corticosteroids ± long acting β-agonist (Advair) preferred
- Leukotriene modifiers (Accolate or Singulair)
- Theophylline
- Mast cell stabilizing agents (cromolyn)
- Additional treatment includes education on exacerbating environmental factors.

▶ CHEST PAIN

RISK FACTORS FOR CORONARY ARTERY DISEASE

- Age
- Hypertension
- DM
- Hyperlipidemia
- Smoking
- Family history of premature coronary artery disease
- Chronic renal insufficiency

DIFFERENTIAL DIAGNOSIS

- GERD
- Angina
- Acute ischemic heart disease
- Aortic dissection
- Acute pericarditis
- Pulmonary embolism

DIAGNOSIS

- ECG findings may include ST-segment elevation.
- Troponins and CK-MB elevated 6–8 hours after onset of chest pain.
- Troponins remain elevated for several days.
- CXR may show evidence of heart failure or enlarged heart.

▶ HYPERTENSION

DIAGNOSIS

- Defined as systolic BP ≥140 mmHg **or** diastolic BP ≥90 mmHg.
- Prehypertension defined as systolic BP 120–139 and diastolic BP 80–89 mmHg.

Major Causes

- Benign essential hypertension
- Secondary hypertension—more likely if early or rapid onset:
  - Renal disease: Renovascular disease, polycystic kidney disease
  - Endocrine: Thyroid, hyperaldosteronism, Cushing syndrome, pheochromocytoma, congenital adrenal hyperplasia
  - Drugs: Oral contraceptives, steroids, NSAIDs, cocaine

Complications

- Long-term hypertension is associated with:
  - Myocardial infarction
  - Heart failure
  - Stroke
  - Renal disease

TREATMENT

- Lifestyle modifications:
  - Sodium restriction
  - Diet and weight reduction
  - Exercise
  - Limit alcohol consumption
- Medical therapy:
  - Diuretics—usually first-line
  - β-Blockers—especially if history of myocardial infarction
  - Calcium channel blockers
  - Angiotensin-converting enzyme inhibitors—recommended in patients with DM, myocardial infarction, or proteinuria

▶ ABDOMINAL PAIN

DIFFERENTIAL DIAGNOSIS

- Cholelithiasis or cholecystitis
- Pancreatitis
- Dyspepsia
- Gastroenteritis

Cholelithiasis and Cholecystitis

- More common in women
- Incidence increases with age

SYMPTOMS

- Cholelithiasis: Biliary colic (crampy right upper quadrant pain), abdominal bloating, dyspepsia
- Cholecystitis: Sudden pain, nausea, vomiting, fever

PHYSICAL EXAMINATION

- Cholelithiasis: Normal physical examination
- Cholecystitis: Right upper quadrant tenderness, guarding, positive Murphy sign (inspiratory arrest with palpation of right upper quadrant), fever, jaundice

LABORATORY AND STUDIES

- Cholelithiasis: Stones on ultrasound
- Cholecystitis:
  - Labs: Leukocytosis, elevated total bilirubin, and transaminases
  - Ultrasound: Gallbladder wall thickening, Murphy sign with transducer
  - HIDA scan: High sensitivity and specificity

TREATMENT

- Cholelithiasis: No treatment if asymptomatic. If symptomatic, consider prophylactic cholecystectomy or expectant management.
- Cholecystitis: Antibiotics if severely ill, bowel rest, cholecystectomy after symptoms resolved.

Pancreatitis

ETIOLOGY

- 80% result from alcohol or gallstones
- Other causes include drugs, metabolic, mass, infectious, hypertriglyceridemia

SYMPTOMS

- Sudden onset, persistent, deep epigastric pain radiating to back
- Pain worsens when patient supine. Improves when sits or leans forward
- Severe nausea, vomiting, fever

PHYSICAL EXAMINATION

- Abdominal tenderness, guarding, rebound
- Distention, ileus, hypotension in severe cases
- Umbilical (Cullen sign) or flank (Grey Turner sign) ecchymosis—rare

LABORATORY AND STUDIES

- Labs: Leukocytosis, elevated amylase (sensitive), elevated lipase (specific), high glucose, elevated AST, ALT
- Abdominal x-ray: Gallstones, sentinel loop (air-filled small bowel in left upper quadrant)
- Ultrasound: Cholelithiasis often present

TREATMENT

- Patient should be kept NPO with aggressive IV hydration
- Pain control with narcotics. Morphine should be avoided as it increases tone of sphincter of Oddi

Dyspepsia

SYMPTOMS

- Localized pain in upper abdomen
- Fullness, bloating, early satiety, nausea, vomiting

DIAGNOSIS

- Based on clinical history and response to empiric treatment
- Endoscopy indicated if any of the following present:
  - Age >50 years, weight loss >10%, melena, anemia
  - Persistent vomiting, hematemesis, dysphagia
  - Abdominal mass, family history of gastric cancer

- Acid suppression with proton pump inhibitors
- If *Helicobacter pylori* present, treat with antibiotics and proton pump inhibitors

▶ GASTROENTERITIS

ETIOLOGY

- Usually viral etiology, with most common causes being:
  - Norovirus (90% of viral gastroenteritis in the United States)
  - Rotavirus
  - Enteric adenovirus
  - Astrovirus

SYMPTOMS

- Incubation period of 24–48 hours
- Nausea, vomiting, diarrhea
- Malaise, fever, myalgia, headache

DIAGNOSIS

- Usually based on clinical symptoms
- Studies may include:
  - Viral serologies
  - Stool culture
  - Stool sample for ova and parasite analysis

TREATMENT

- Usually symptomatic relief, hydration
- If severe dehydration occurs, may require IV hydration

▶ URINARY TRACT INFECTIONS

Definitions

- Urethritis: Inflammation of urethra. Symptoms of dysuria and frequency.
- Cystitis: Inflammation of bladder. Symptoms same as urethritis.
- Bacteriuria: Presence of bacteria in bladder. Defined as infection if:
  - $\geq 10^2$ colony-forming units per milliliter (cfu/mL) with symptoms
  - $\geq 10^5$ cfu/mL and asymptomatic
- Urethral syndrome: Frequency, urgency, dysuria, suprapubic discomfort, and voiding difficulties in absence of organic pathology. Diagnosis of exclusion.

Pathogenesis

- Hematogenous, lymphatic spread, or ascending extension. Organisms involved:
  - *Escherichia coli* (80%)
  - *Streptococcus saprophyticus* (10–15%)
  - *Klebsiella* (5%)
  - *Enterobacter* and *Proteus* (2%)
- *Serratia marcescens* and *Pseudomonas aeruginosa* almost always in hospitalized patients, associated with urethral catheterization.
- Predisposing factors are sexual intercourse, diaphragm use, recent urinary tract infection (UTI), systemic illness, urinary tract catheterization, and anomalies.

DIAGNOSIS

- Clean-catch or catheterized specimen for microscopy or urine culture.
- IV pyelogram (IVP) indicated if:
  - History of prior upper UTI, recurrent UTIs, or childhood UTIs
  - Painless hematuria
  - History of stones or obstruction
- Rapid recurrence is suspicious for bacterial persistence or presence of fistula (enterovesical, vesicovaginal).
- Voiding cystourethrogram if suspect urethral diverticulum.

TREATMENT

- Hydration, acidify urine to prevent recurrent infections.
- Analgesics (i.e., Pyridium) used only for 2–3 days.
- Cranberry juice may inhibit bacterial adherence.
- Empiric therapy for acute uncomplicated cystitis include:
  - TMP-SMX
  - Nitrofurantoin
- Quinoline (in areas of known resistance to TMP-SMX or in complicated UTIs).
- Asymptomatic bacteriuria during pregnancy should be treated.
- Asymptomatic bacteriuria in elderly, diabetics, spinal cord injury patients do not require screening or treatment.

Pyelonephritis

- Inflammation of kidney and renal pelvis
- Associated with fever, chills, costovertebral angle tenderness
- If no comorbidities: Treat as outpatient with 14-day course of fluoroquinolone
- If no improvement in 72 hours: Should reevaluate, image, consider obstruction.

▶ HEADACHES

Tension Headache

SYMPTOMS

- Pressure, tightness all around head
- Usually devoid of associated symptoms

- Normal neurological examination

- Therapy at time of onset:
  - Acetaminophen
  - Aspirin
  - NSAIDs
- Prophylactic therapy if requiring daily analgesics:
  - Tricyclic antidepressants
  - Behavioral therapy
- If neurological symptoms present or no relief with conventional treatment, should consider imaging or referral to specialist

Migraine Headache

- Most patients are young, women
- 90% have strong family history

- Recurrent headaches, with episodes lasting 4–72 hours
- Classically unilateral, pulsating pain
- Associated with photophobia, phonophobia, anorexia, nausea, vomiting
- May have preceding aura (20%) or focal neurological deficit (migraine variant)

- Normal neurological examination.
- If focal neurological deficits present, imaging workup (CT, MRI), required.

- Therapy at time of migraine onset:
  - Triptans
  - Ergotamine (should be avoided in vascular disease or pregnant patients)
  - Acetaminophen/butalbital/caffeine (i.e., Fioricet)
  - Antiemetics (prochlorperazine, promethazine)
- Prophylactic therapy if frequent, severe migraines:
  - Tricyclic antidepressants or SSRIs
  - β-Blockers
  - Calcium channel blockers
  - Antiseizure medication
- If neurological symptoms present or no relief with conventional treatment, should consider imaging or referral to specialist

Cluster Headache

- Classically in young men
- Family history not often seen

SYMPTOMS

- Occurs 2–3 times daily over several weeks, lasting 30 minutes to 2 hours
- Abrupt onset, severe, unilateral "ice pick–like" periorbital pain
- Associated with ipsilateral autonomic symptoms (i.e., tearing of the eye and nares)
- Onset with sleep or alcohol very characteristic

PHYSICAL EXAMINATION

- Restless, agitated, often pacing the room
- May find tearing, nasal discharge, ptosis on ipsilateral side
- No focal neurological deficits

TREATMENT

- Therapy at time of onset:
  - Oxygen inhalation is most effective treatment (5–10 L/min for 10–15 minutes)
  - Intranasal lidocaine ointment
  - Triptans (see Migraine Headaches)
- Prophylactic therapy
  - Verapamil
  - Prednisone taper at beginning of cluster
  - Lithium
  - Valproate
- If neurological symptoms present or no relief with conventional treatment, should consider imaging or referral to specialist.

Sinus-Related Headache

SYMPTOMS

- Purulence in nasal cavity
- Facial pain, pressure, congestion, fullness
- Nasal obstruction, blockage, discharge, purulence
- Hyposmia or anosmia

PHYSICAL EXAMINATION

- Normal neurological examination
- Sinus tenderness
- Nasal discharge or blockage

TREATMENT

- Nasal corticosteroids or antihistamines
- If infection present, should treat with antibiotics
- If neurological symptoms present or no relief with treatment, should consider imaging or referral to specialist on an urgent basis as there is increased risk of brain abscess or subdural or epidural empyema in presence of chronic sinusitis.

Headache Due to Central Nervous System Anomaly

ANEURYSM

- Typically causes headache when ruptures, leading to subarachnoid hemorrhage.
- Giant aneurysms can cause headache even without rupture.
- Severe headache with sudden onset.
- Classically described as "worst headache of their life."
- Decreased level of consciousness, photophobia, and stiff neck may be present.
- Diagnosis of subarachnoid hemorrhage made with noncontrast head CT. Lumbar puncture is gold standard and is indicated if CT negative.
- Requires immediate workup and treatment due to high risk of morbidity and mortality within the first 24 hours if untreated.

ARTERIOVENOUS MALFORMATION

- Usually present with intracranial hemorrhage or seizures.
- Angiography is gold standard for diagnosis.

TUMOR

- Uncommon cause of headaches.
- Headaches occur in 50% of patients with brain tumor.
- Symptoms may worsen with bending over, or coughing, sneezing, Valsalva.
- Nausea, vomiting, neurological symptoms may be present.

▶ PSYCHIATRIC DISORDERS

Depression

RISK FACTORS

- Family history
- Lifetime prevalence twice as high in women (20% in women, 10% in men)

SIGNS AND SYMPTOMS

- Five of the following symptoms, one of which must be either depressed mood or anhedonia:
    - Depressed mood
    - Anhedonia (loss of pleasure)
    - Hypersomnia or insomnia
    - Feelings of guilt
    - Decreased energy or fatigue
    - Decreased concentration
    - Decreased appetite
    - Suicidal ideation
    - Psychomotor agitation or retardation
    - Significant change in weight
- Severely depressed patients can develop psychotic symptoms.

Anxiety Disorder

SIGNS AND SYMPTOMS

- Symptoms must interfere with social or occupational functioning
- Chronic baseline anxiety, not just when exposed to a trigger.
- At least three of the following symptoms must be present:
    - Restlessness
    - Poor concentration
    - Irritability
    - Easy fatigue
    - Muscle tension
    - Sleep disturbances

Psychosis

SIGNS AND SYMPTOMS

- Delusions: Fixed false beliefs
- Hallucinations: Auditory, visual, tactile
- Disorganized thought: Disruption of logical thought process

Bipolar Affective Disorder

SIGNS AND SYMPTOMS

- Extreme mood swings between mania and depression.
- In severe phases of mania or depression, patients can have psychotic symptoms.

Panic Disorder

SIGNS AND SYMPTOMS

- Panic attacks must include ≥4 of the following:
    - Tachycardia
    - Diaphoresis
    - Shortness of breath
    - Chest pain
    - Nausea
    - Dizziness
    - Paresthesias
    - Chills
    - Fear of losing control or dying
- Abrupt development of above symptoms that peak within 10 minutes
- With or without agoraphobia

Obsessive Compulsive Disorder

SIGNS AND SYMPTOMS

- Symptoms cause significant impairment and are excessive or unreasonable.
- Obsessions are recurrent or persistent thoughts that cause anxiety.
- Compulsions are behaviors or rituals that temporarily decrease anxiety.

- Patients must recognize that their symptoms are unreasonable (if not, then likely delusional disorder)
  - Tachycardia
  - Diaphoresis

Contact Dermatitis

- Result of direct skin contact to irritant or allergen

SIGNS AND SYMPTOMS

- Erythema, chapped skin, dryness, fissuring
- Mild to extreme itching
- Severe cases may result in edema, oozing, pain, or bullae
- Poison ivy, poison oak, and poison sumac are all types of irritant dermatitis:
  - Symptoms usually develop within 4–96 hours of exposure.
  - Blister fluid is not antigenic.
  - Most common complication is bacterial infection of skin with *Staphylococcus aureus*.

TREATMENT

- Restore normal epidermal barrier
- Prevent contact to irritant or allergen
- Topical corticosteroids may be useful in severe, acute phase

Eczema (Atopic Dermatitis)

- Familial, with allergic features
- Often in patients who have asthma and allergic rhinitis

SIGNS AND SYMPTOMS

- Scaling, crusting, oozing
- Intense itching
- Erythematous patches, vesicles, and exudates

TREATMENT

- Minimizing exposure to potential allergens
- Emollients
- Antihistamines
- Topical corticosteroids
- Elidel or protopic
- Refer to dermatology for consideration of oral immunosuppressants

Seborrheic Dermatitis

SIGNS AND SYMPTOMS

- Erythema (pink-red)
- Scaliness
- Mild itching

TREATMENT

- If on the scalp, treatment with tar, selenium, or zinc shampoo
- If not on scalp, treatment with topical corticosteroids or antifungal agents

Acne

- Most common cutaneous disorder in the United States
- Factors involved are:
    - Retention hyperkeratosis
    - Increased sebum production
    - Presence of Propionibacterium acnes
    - Inflammation

SIGNS AND SYMPTOMS

- Usually affects face, neck, chest, upper back, upper arms.
- May include blackheads, whiteheads, or inflammatory lesions

TREATMENT

- Topical retinoids (tretinoin, adapalene)
- Oral isotretinonin (Accutane)
- Salicylic acid, glycolic acid
- Benzoyl peroxide
- Topical antibiotics (erythromycin, clindamycin, tetracycline)
- Oral antibiotics (tetracycline, doxycycline, minocycline, erythromycin, clindamycin)

Basal Cell Carcinoma

- Accounts for 80% of all skin cancers

SIGNS AND SYMPTOMS

- Papules or nodules with telangiectasias and **pearly** quality.
- Often find a central erosion or crust.
- Lesions on chest or back will often be scaly and erythematous (may resemble eczema).

TREATMENT

- Depends on tumor and patient.
- Treatment may be surgical or nonsurgical.

Squamous Cell Carcinoma

- Typically affects patients >55 years

SIGNS AND SYMPTOMS

- Usually in areas exposed to the sun (head, neck, hands, forearms, legs)
- Firm, hyperkeratotic papules, plaques, or nodules
- Poorly differentiated and may have ulcerations, hemorrhage, or necrosis

Squamous cell carcinoma of the skin is the most common cancer in women 25–29 years old.

TREATMENT

- Surgical excision recommended

Melanoma

- Most prevalent cancer in women 25–29 years old

SIGNS AND SYMPTOMS

- May occur on any skin or mucosal surface.
- Findings that may signify malignancy of a mole ("ABCDE"):
  - Asymmetric
  - Borders are irregular
  - Color variegation
  - Diameter >6 mm
  - Enlargement

TREATMENT

- Excision
- Sentinel lymph node dissection if melanoma >1 mm thick
- Possible adjuvant therapy

▶ DIABETES MELLITUS

Classification

- Type 1 DM:
  - Associated with genetic predisposition
  - Caused by autoimmune destruction of pancreatic islet cells
- Type 2 DM:
  - Strong polygenic predisposition
  - Due to insulin resistance

RISK FACTORS

- Type 2 DM:
  - Family history
  - Obese
  - Personal history of gestational diabetes
  - Increased incidence in certain ethnic groups: Latinos, Asian/Pacific Islanders, African Americans, Native Americans

SIGNS AND SYMPTOMS

- The three "polys": Polyuria, polydipsia, polyphagia
- May present with vulvovaginitis, rapid weight loss, dehydration, blurry vision, neuropathy

DIAGNOSIS

- Physical examination should be done to assess for end organ damage:
  - Ophthalmological examination to assess retinopathy
  - Cardiovascular examination to assess atherosclerosis
  - Neurological examination to assess neuropathy

- Any one of the following is diagnostic:
  - Symptoms and a random glucose ≥200 mg/dL
  - Fasting glucose ≥126 mg/dL on two separate occasions
  - 2-hour post-Glucola (75 g load) glucose ≥200 mg/dL

TREATMENT

- Initial attempt to control with diet and exercise
- Oral medications, usually start with single agent, then add as needed:
  - Sulfonylureas (Glipizide, Glyburide)
  - Biguanide (metformin)
  - Thiazolidinediones (rosiglitazone, pioglitazone)
  - α-Glucosidase inhibitors (acarbose)
- Injectable medications, to supplement or replace oral agents as necessary
  - Exenatide (beretta)
  - Insulin

▶ THYROID DISEASES

Hypothyroidism

CAUSES

- Hashimoto's (autoimmune) thyroiditis:
  - Most common cause in the United States
- Subacute thyroiditis
- Drugs
  - Amiodarone, lithium, interferon, iodide
- Iatrogenic
  - Postsurgical, postradioactive iodine treatment
- Iodine deficiency
  - Rare in the United States, but common worldwide

SIGNS AND SYMPTOMS

- Fatigue, weight gain, cold intolerance
- Dry skin, menstrual irregularities, constipation

DIAGNOSIS

- Physical examination findings may include:
  - Periorbital edema, peripheral edema
  - Bradycardia, hoarse voice, coarse hair
  - Thyroid may be small or enlarged
- ECG may show low voltage.
- Laboratory tests most commonly show:
  - Elevated TSH
  - Decreased free T_4
  - Positive TPO antibodies may be found in Hashimoto's

TREATMENT

- Thyroid hormone replacement

Hyperthyroidism

CAUSES

- Graves disease
- Solitary toxic nodule
- Multinodular goiter
- Thyroiditis

SIGNS AND SYMPTOMS

- Weight loss, anxiety, palpitations, fatigue, hyperdefecation
- Heat intolerance, sweating, amenorrhea

DIAGNOSIS

- Physical examination findings may include:
  - Lid lag, tachycardia, hyperreflexia
  - Diffuse or multinodular goiter
- Graves disease patients may also have:
  - Exophthalmos, proptosis, periorbital edema, pretibial myxedema
  - Onycholysis very specific for Graves disease
- Laboratory tests commonly show:
  - Decreased TSH
  - Elevated free T_4 and free T_3
  - Thyroglobulin, TPO antibodies, and TSI
- Radioactive iodine scan indicated if type of hyperthyroidism in question or if radioactive iodine therapy planned.

TREATMENT

- Decrease thyroid hormone production:
  - Methimazole blocks thyroid hormone formation only.
  - Propylthiouracil (PTU) blocks thyroid hormone formation and peripheral conversion.
- Radioactive iodine is first choice for toxic nodule or Graves disease.
- Surgery if uncontrolled disease during pregnancy or if unable to perform radioactive iodine.
- β-Blockers can be used in acute phase for tachycardia.

▶ ARTHRITIS

DIFFERENTIAL DIAGNOSIS

- Osteoarthritis—exacerbated by activity and relieved with rest
- Rheumatoid arthritis—improved with activity. Morning pain and stiffness common
- Infectious arthritis—bacterial nongonococcal, gonococcal, viral, or fungal
- Gout—recurrent attacks of inflammatory arthritis caused by monosodium urate crystals. Associated with hyperuricemia
- Psoriatic arthritis

SIGNS AND SYMPTOMS

- Pain aggravated by movement
- Loss of motion
- Swelling

DIAGNOSIS

- X-ray may help identify joint effusion that may not be evident on examination.
- Synovial fluid aspiration—can differentiate if joint effusion is:
  - Inflammatory
  - Infected
  - Bloody
  - Containing urate cystals (hallmark of gout)
- Laboratory tests
  - ANA has high sensitivity, but low specificity for systemic lupus erythematosus.
  - Rheumatoid factor should be ordered if clinical suspicion of rheumatoid arthritis. Has low sensitivity and low specificity.

TREATMENT OF OSTEOARTHRITIS

- Nonpharmacological therapy:
  - Weight loss
  - Rest for short periods of time
  - Exercise and physical therapy
- Pharmacological therapy:
  - Acetaminophen
  - NSAIDs
  - Intraarticular glucocorticosteroids
  - Glucosamine and chondroitin

▶ LOW BACK PAIN

- 80% will have at least one episode of acute back pain in their lifetime.
- Acute low back pain is most common musculoskeletal problem of women.

DIFFERENTIAL DIAGNOSIS

- Muscle strain (spasm of paravertebral muscles)
- Mechanical: Osteoarthritis, spinal stenosis, spondylolisthesis, compression fracture
- Infection: Epidural abscess, vertebral osteomyelitis, diskitis
- Inflammatory arthritis: Rheumatoid arthritis, ankylosing spondylitis
- Tumor: Metastasis, multiple myeloma, lymphoma

History

- If there is no radicular pain, it is unlikely to be disc herniation.
- Sciatic pain in the **lower** leg may be indicative of nerve root irritation.
- Atypical presentation which would warrant referral:
  - Weight loss, history of carcinoma, trauma, unrelenting pain
  - Saddle anesthesia, bowel or bladder incontinence warrant immediate neurosurgery referral (cauda equina syndrome)

DIAGNOSIS

- Physical examination is of limited value. Should include:
  - Straight leg raise in supine position (positive test is sign of herniated lumbar disc).
  - Detailed neurological examination to elicit hypoesthesia or hyperesthesia.
- MRI and CT both have poor sensitivity and specificity

TREATMENT OF MUSCLE STRAIN

- Conservative treatment for 6–8 weeks usually resolves symptoms.
- Rest, with limitation of activity helps decrease acute pain.
- Medical therapy:
  - NSAIDs
  - Muscle relaxants
  - Narcotics
- Local thermal therapy (heating pads, ice packs, whirlpool).
- Benefit of low back exercises is controversial.

INDEX

biophysical profile, 25–26
bipolar disorder, 216
    risk in pregnancy, 77
    symptoms of, 77
    treatment of, 77
BI-RADS. *See* Breast Imaging Reporting
    and Data System
Bishop scoring system, 32*t*
blastocyte, 8*f*
    formation of, 9*f*
blues, postpartum, 44
BRCA mutations, 163
breach of standard care, 201
breast abscess, 115
breast cancer, 163–167
    diagnosis of, 164–166
    epidemiology of, 163
    pathology of, 165
    pregnancy and, 166–167
    prognostic factors, 165–166
    risk factors for, 163–164
    treatment of, 166
Breast Imaging Reporting and Data
    System (BI-RADS), 164
breastfeeding, 41
bronchitis, 205–206
    diagnosis of, 206
    differential diagnosis of, 206
    signs and symptoms of, 205
    treatment of, 206

C

Call-Exner bodies, 169
cancer, staging of, 187–188
candidiasis, 102
carbamazepine, 28
carbon dioxide, 126
carcinoma. *See specific types*
cardiac disease, 15
cardiogenic shock, 124
cardiovascular disease, 64–67
    common, 65–67
    diagnostic evaluation of, 64–65
cardiovascular system
    in pregnancy, 10–11
    in puerperium, 42
case control studies, 197
cell cycle, 161
central monitoring, 124
central venous pressure monitoring, 124
cervical incompetence, second
    trimester loss and, 80
cervical neoplasia, 171–174
    diagnosis of, 172
    epidemiology of, 171
    human papillomavirus and, 172
    pathology of, 172
    pregnancy and, 174
    risk factors for, 171–172

staging of, 172, 187, 189*t*
    treatment of, 172–173, 174*t*
cervix
    in normal labor, 29
    in puerperium, 40
Cesarian delivery, 35
chancroid, 103–104
chemotherapy, 162
    common agents, 162*t*
chest pain, 208
    diagnosis of, 208
    differential diagnosis of, 208
    risk factors for, 208
chest x-ray, 65
chlamydia, 102
    diagnosis of, 58
    fetal effects of, 58
    signs and symptoms of, 58
cholecystitis, 209
    effects of, on pregnancy, 69
    symptoms and diagnosis of, 69, 209
    treatment of, 69, 210
cholestasis
    effects of, on pregnancy, 70
    symptoms and diagnosis of, 70
    treatment of, 70
cholesterol testing, 201
cholelithiasis, 69, 209
    symptoms and diagnosis of, 69, 209
    treatment of, 69, 210
choriocarcinoma, 169, 184–185
    diagnosis of, 184
    symptoms of, 184
    treatment of, 184–185
chorionic villi, 13
    sampling of, 24
chronic hypothalamic anovulation, 143
chronic pelvic pain, 113–114
    differential diagnosis, 113–114
chronic retention of urine, 111
circumcision, infant, 39
claims made policy, 200
Clomid. *See* clomiphene citrate
clomiphene citrate (Clomid), 154,
    155–156
cocaine, 27
cohort studies, 197
coitus interruptus, 127
collagen, loss of, 157
collagen vascular disorders, 74–77
colorectal cancer screening, 201–202
colporrhaphy, 108
condom, male, 127
condyloma acuminatum, 104
contact dermatitis, 217
contraception, 127–130, 139
    definitions of, 127
    failure rates of, 128*t*
    methods of, 127–130
    in puerperium, 42

contraceptive patch, 129
contraceptive vaginal ring, 129
contraction-stress test (CST), 25
copper intrauterine device, 129
core-needle biopsy, 165
coronary artery disease, 157, 208
corpus luteum cyst, 112
critical care, 123–124
cross-sectional study, 198
CST. *See* contraction-stress test
current health status, preconceptual
    counseling and, 14–15
Cushing syndrome, 73–74
    management of, 74
    pregnancy and, 73
    symptoms and diagnosis of, 73
cyst
    Bartholin gland, 105–106
    of the canal of nuck, 106
    corpus luteum, 112
    epidermal inclusion, 105
    functional ovarian, 112
    sebaceous, 105
    theca lutein, 112
cytomegalovirus, 54–55
    diagnosis of, 54–55
    fetal effects of, 55
    prevention of, 55
    signs and symptoms of, 54
cytotrophoblasts, 9

D

death, leading causes of, 201
decidua basalis, 141
decidua functionalis, 141
decision analysis, 198
deep vein thrombosis, 63–64
    anticoagulation in pregnancy, 63
    causes of, 63
    diagnosis, 63
    peripartum management of, 64
    treatment, 63
dehiscence, postpartum, 43
depot medroxyprogesterone acetate
    (DMPA), 129
depression
    postpartum, 44–45
    risk factors for, 215
    risk in pregnancy, 78
    symptoms of, 78, 215
    treatment of, 78, 158
dermatological disorders, 94–96,
    217–219
DES. *See* diethylstilbestrol
Dextran. *See* Hyskon
DHT. *See* dihydrotestosterone
diabetes, 219–220. *See* gestational dia-
    betes; pregestational diabetes
    classification of, 219

diagnosis of, 219–220
risk factors for, 219
signs and symptoms of, 219
treatment of, 219–220
diabetic ketoacidosis, 50–51
diaphragm (contraception), 128
diethylstilbestrol (DES), 28–29
diffuse papillomatosis, 116
dihydrotestosterone (DHT), 135
DMPA. *See* depot medroxyprogesterone acetate
DNR indications. *See* Do not
resuscitate indications
Do not resuscitate (DNR)
indications, 187
Donovanosis. *See* granuloma inguinale
doppler velocimetry, 26
drugs, 26–29
recreational, 26–27
ductus venosus, 13
dysgerminoma, 168
dysmenorrhea, 138, 141–142
diagnosis of, 142
primary, 141
risk factors for, 142
secondary, 141
treatment of, 142
dyspareunia, 132
dyspepsia, 210–211
diagnosis of, 211
symptoms of, 210
treatment of, 211

E

eating disorders, 78
risk in pregnancy, 78
symptoms of, 78
treatment of, 78
echocardiography, 65
economic analysis, 198
ectopic pregnancy, 118–119
counseling, 119
diagnosis of, 118
risk factors for, 118
treatment of, 118–119
eczema, 105, 217
electrocardiogram, 64
embryology, 8–10
anatomy and, 161–163
embryonic development, 8–9
fertilization, 8
gametogenesis, 8
embryonal carcinoma, 169
embryonic development
singleton, 8–10
twin gestation, 10
empty sella syndrome, 144
endocrine disorders, 72–74, 120
endodermal sinus, 168

endometrial cancer, 174–176
characteristics of, 174t
diagnosis of, 175
histology of, 175–176
risk factors for, 174
screening for, 175
survival rates for, 176
treatment of, 176
endometrial carcinoma, 175–176
treatment of, 176
endometrial hyperplasia, 175
treatment of, 176
endometrial polyp, 101
endometrioma, 113
endometriosis, 114–115
diagnostic tests, 114
pathogenesis of, 114
physical findings in, 114
staging system, 114
symptoms of, 114
treatment of, 114–115
endometritis, postpartum, 42
endometrium, menstrual cycle and,
141
epidemiology, errors in, 199
epidermal inclusion cysts, 105
epidural anesthesia, 37
epilepsy, 16
episiotomy
infection and dehiscence, 43
median, 35
mediolateral, 35
epithelial ovarian cancer, 168
treatment of, 170–171
estrogens, 28, 163
ethics, 196
ethnicity, 16–17
heritable diseases and, 20t
excisional biopsy, 165
exercise, prenatal care and, 19
expanded MS-AFP, 23–24
eye infection, 39

F

fallopian tube, 162
fallopian tube cancer, 181
diagnosis of, 181
histology of, 181
staging of, 181, 188
treatment and survival of, 181
family history, 16
fasting glucose testing, 202
fat necrosis, 115–116
female sexual differentiation, 135
fertilization, 8
fetal circulation, 13, 13f
fetal death
complications of, 94
diagnosis of, 93

fetal causes of, 92
maternal causes of, 92–93
placental causes of, 92
fever, 122
fibroadenoma, 115
fibrocystic disease, 115
fibroids, 101
fibromas, 106, 113
fibronectin, 82
fine needle aspiration, 164–165
first trimester pregnancy loss, 116–118,
117
definitions of, 116
diagnosis of, 117
etiology of, 116–117
risk factors for, 117
statistics, 117
fluoxetine, 79
folic acid deficiency, 60–61
causes of, 60
diagnosis of, 61
effects of, on fetus, 61
treatment of, 61
follicular phase, 140
forceps, 35t
functional hypothalamic amenorrhea,
143
functional ovarian cyst, 112

G

galactocele, 115
gametogenesis, 8
gastroenteritis, 211
diagnosis of, 211
etiology of, 211
symptoms of, 211
treatment of, 211
gastrointestinal disease, 68–70
gastrointestinal tract, pregnancy and,
11–12
GBS. *See* group B streptococci
general anesthesia, 37
genetic counseling, 20–23
aneuploidy, 21
autosomal dominant, 20
autosomal recessive, 21
common genetic disorders, 22–23
indications for, 23
multifactorial inheritance, 21
structural abnormalities, 21–22
triploidy, 22
x-linked diseases, 21
genital herpes. *See* herpes simplex
virus
genital tract, pregnancy and, 10, 11t
geriatric patient care, 125
functional assessment, 125
preventive health services, 125
surgical care, 125

Müllerian tract development, 135–136
multifactorial inheritance, 21
multifetal reduction, 88
multiple gestations, 86–88
    complications of, 87–88
    diagnosis of, 86
    fetal risks of, 87
    intrauterine demise of fetus in, 88
    management of, 87
    maternal risks of, 87
    monoamniotic twin gestation and, 88
    multifetal reduction and, 88
    risk factors for, 86
    twin-twin transfusion syndrome and,
        87–88
multiple sclerosis, 72
    pregnancy and, 72
    symptoms of, 72
muscle strain, 223
myasthenia gravis
    pregnancy and, 71
    symptoms of, 71

N

naloxone, 36
natural family planning, 127
negligent tort, 201
neonatal evaluation, 37
    algorithm for, 38f
neonatal resuscitation, 38–40
    eye infection prophylaxis, 39
    infant circumcision, 39
    umbilical cord blood gases, 39
neoplasia. *See also specific types*
nephrolithiasis, 51–52
    diagnosis of, 52
    effects of, on pregnancy, 52
    symptoms of, 51
    treatment of, 52
nephrotic syndrome, 52
    diagnosis of, 52
    effects of, on pregnancy, 52
    treatment of, 52
neural tube defects, 16
neurological diseases, 70–72
    diagnosis of, 70
non-stress test (NST), 25
normal saline (NS), 126
NS. *See* normal saline
NST. *See* non-stress test
nutrition, prenatal care and, 18

O

obesity, 14
obsessive compulsive disorder, 78,
    216–217
    risk in pregnancy, 78
    symptoms of, 78
    treatment of, 78

obstetric anesthesia, 35–37
obstetric screening, 23–25
    amniocentesis, 25
    chorionic villus sampling, 24
    diagnostic tests, 24–25
    expanded MS-AFP, 23–24
    first trimester, 23
    tests, 23
obstruction, 122
occurrence policy, 200
odds ratio, 197t
oligomenorrhea, 138
oncogenes, 161
oncology
    genetics and, 161
    pain management, 186–187
    pharmacology and
        chemotherapy, 162
    physiology and, 161
oocytes, 8
oogonia, 8
operative delivery, 34–35
oral contraceptives, 128–129
orgasm, 131
osteoarthritis, 222
osteoporosis, 157
    treatment of, 158
otitis media, 204
    diagnosis of, 204
    signs and symptoms of, 204
    treatment of, 204
ovarian cancer, 167–171
    diagnosis of, 167, 170
    epithelial, 168
    familial syndromes, 167
    histology of, 168–170
    low malignant potential, 169–170
    screening for, 167
    staging of, 167, 188, 190t–191t
    treatment of, 170–171
ovarian cycle, 8f
ovarian disease, 142–143
    treatment for, 147
ovarian hyperthecosis, 142
ovarian masses, 111–113, 138
    diagnostic studies, 111–112
    differential diagnosis of, 112–113
    history, 111
    physical exam, 111
ovary, 161
overactive bladder, 110–111
ovulation induction agents,
    155–156
ovulation, puerperium and, 40–41

P

Paget disease, 165, 177
pain management, 186–187
palliative care, 187

pancreatitis
    etiology of, 210
    laboratory and studies on, 210
    physical examination of, 210
    symptoms of, 69, 210
    treatment of, 69, 210
panic disorder, 216
paracervical block, 36
parathyroid disorders, 74
paravaginal repair, 108
parenteral (IV) analgesia, 35–36
paroxetine, 79
parvovirus, 54
    diagnosis of, 54
    fetal effects of, 54
    symptoms of, 54
patient education, prenatal care and,
    18–19
PCOS. *See* polycystic ovary syndrome
PCP. *See* phencyclidine
pediatric gynecology, 136–139
pelvic muscle exercise, 107
pelvic pain, 138
pelvic support defects, 106–109
    causes of, 107
    evaluation of, 107
    treatment of, 107–109
pelvic types, 30f, 30t
    mnemonic for, 31
pemphigoid gestationis. *See* herpes
    gestationis
periodic health assessment, 201–204
perioperative care, 121–123
peripheral artery cannulation, 124
periurethral injection, 110
pessary, 107
phencyclidine (PCP), 27
phenobarbital, 28
phenytoin, 27–28
pheochromocytoma
    management of, 73
    pregnancy and, 73
    symptoms and diagnosis of, 73
pituitary disorders, 74, 144
    treatment for, 147
placenta previa, 83
    diagnosis of, 83
    management of, 83
    recurrence of, 83
    risk factors for, 83
placental abruption, 82–83
    diagnosis of, 82–83
    management of, 83
    recurrence of, 83
    risk factors for, 82
placental site trophoblastic tumor, 185
    diagnosis of, 185
    symptoms of, 185
    treatment of, 185
platypelloid pelvis, 30f, 30t

respiratory system
  complications, 122
  in pregnancy, 12t
respiratory tract infections, 205–207
  upper, 205
retinoids, 28
retropubic suspension, 110
Rhesus blood group system, 90
rheumatoid arthritis, 76–77
  effects of, on pregnancy, 77
  fetal effects of, 77
  management of, 77
  pathophysiology of, 76
  signs and symptoms of, 77
risk management, 200–201
routine screening, 201–203
rubella, 15, 54
  diagnosis of, 54
  fetal effects of, 54
  prevention of, 54
  signs and symptoms, 54

S

sacral colpopexy, 108
sacrospinous fixation, 108
sarcoma, 170
  treatment of, 171
schizophrenia, 77–78
  symptoms of, 77
  treatment of, 78
sclerosing adenosis, 116
sebaceous cysts, 105
seborrheic dermatitis, 217–218
second trimester loss, 79–81
  antiphospholipid antibody syndrome
    and, 80
  causes of, 79–80
  cervical incompetence and, 80
  clinical manifestation of, 79
  diagnosis of, 80–81
  hypothyroidism and, 80
  management of, 81
  recurrence and prevention of, 81
  septate uterus and, 80
seizure disorder, 71
  effects of, on pregnancy, 71
self-payment, 199–200
semen analysis reference values, 155t
sensitivity, 198–199
septate uterus, second trimester loss
    and, 80
septic shock, 123
Sertoli-Leydig tumors, 169
sertraline, 79
serum alpha fetoprotein, abnormal
    maternal, 24t
sexual abuse, 138, 139
sexual differentiation, 135
  females, 135
    males, 135

sexual function disorders, 131–132
sexuality, 131–132
  stages of response, 131
sexually transmitted diseases,
    102–104
Sheehan syndrome, 144
sickle cell disease, 61
  causes of, 61
  diagnosis of, 61
  effects of, 61
  treatment of, 61
skin, pregnancy and, 13
smoking, prenatal care and, 19
SNRI, 79
sorbitol, 126
specificity, 198–199
sperm, 8
spinal anesthesia, 36
squamous cell carcinoma, 177,
    218–219
  survival rates of, 180t
  treatment of, 180t
squamous cell hyperplasia, 105
SSRIs, 79
standard of care, 200
sterilization, 129
stress urinary incontinence (SUI),
    109–110
stromal tumors, 169
  treatment of, 171
structural abnormalities, 21–22
substance abuse, 14
suburethral sling, 110
SUI. See stress urinary incontinence
sulfonamides, 29
Swan-Ganz catheter, 124
syncytiotrophoblasts, 9
syphilis, 57, 103
  diagnosis of, 57
  fetal effects of, 57
  prevention of, 57
  signs and symptoms of, 57
syringoma, 106
systemic lupus erythematosus,
    74–75
  diagnosis of, 75
  fetal effects of, 75
  management of, 75
  maternal effects of, 75
  pathophysiology of, 74
  signs and symptoms of, 74

T

tail coverage, 200
TCA, 79
teratogenicity, 26
teratoma, 169
testosterone, 135
tetanus vaccination, 204
tetracycline, 29

β-thalassemia minor, 61–62
  causes of, 61
diagnosis of, 61
  effects of, on fetus, 62
  treatment of, 62
theca lutein cyst, 112
third trimester bleeding, 82–84
  genital tract abnormalities
    and, 84
  labor and, 84
thrombocytopenia, 62
  causes of, 62
  diagnosis of, 62
  effects of, on fetus, 62
  treatment of, 62
thromboembolism, 122
  postpartum, 44
thrombophilias, 16
  acquired, 120
  inherited, 120–121
thrombotic thrombocytopenic purpura,
    62–63
  causes of, 62
  diagnosis, 63
  effects of, on fetus, 63
  treatment, 63
thyroid
  disorders, 72–73, 220–221
  in pregnancy, 12–13
tobacco, 27
topoisomerase inhibitors, 162
toxic shock syndrome, 123
toxoplasmosis, 15
  diagnosis of, 55
  fetal effects of, 55
  prevention of, 55
  signs and symptoms of, 55
translocation, 22
transverse vaginal septum, 144
trauma, 138
travel, prenatal care and, 19
trial of labor, 34
trichomonas vaginalis, 102
triploidy, 22
trisomy 13, 23
trisomy 18, 23
trisomy 21, 22
tuberculosis, 68
  fetal effects of, 68
  management of, 68
  skin testing, 203
  symptoms and diagnosis of, 68, 206
  treatment of, 207
tubular adenoma, 116
tumor suppressor genes, 161
Turner syndrome, 23
twin gestation
  dizygotic, 10
  monozygotic, 10
twin-twin transfusion syndrome, 87–88